2 x
27

Health Care Facility Planning & Construction

Health Care Facility Planning & Construction

Burton R. Klein, MSE
Albert J. Platt, ACA

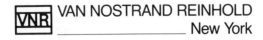 VAN NOSTRAND REINHOLD
New York

Library of Congress Catalog Card Number 88-39810
ISBN 0-442-31847-2

Printed in the United States of America

Van Nostrand Reinhold
115 Fifth Avenue
New York, New York 10003

Van Nostrand Reinhold International Company Limited
11 New Fetter Lane
London EC4P 4EE, England

Van Nostrand Reinhold
480 La Trobe Street
Melbourne, Victoria 3000, Australia

Macmillan of Canada
Division of Canada Publishing Corporation
164 Commander Boulevard
Agincourt, Ontario M1S 3C7, Canada

16 15 14 13 12 11 10 9 8 7 6 5 4 3 2 1

Library of Congress Cataloging-in-Publication Data
Klein, Burton R.
    Health care facility planning and construction / Burton R. Klein,
Albert Platt.
        p. cm.
    Bibliography: p.
    Includes index.
    ISBN 0-442-31847-2 (soft)
    1. Health facilities — Design and construction.   I. Platt, Albert.
II. Title.
    [DNLM: 1. Facility Design and Construction.   WX 140 K64h]
RA967.K543 1989
362.1′1′0682 — dc19
DNLM/DLC
for Library of Congress   88-39810

This book is dedicated to our wives
SANDY and ALICE
for their patience during the several years it has
taken us to produce this book

Contents

Preface

This book has been developed so that those involved in designing, building, and operating health care facilities can understand and appreciate all the work required to produce a facility that will be as reasonably safe as possible for staff to work in and for patients to be treated and housed in. The book provides the fundamentals of the process to achieve a viable facility to meet this objective.

The process of building or renovating a health care facility is very complicated. It involves the coordination of many groups and agencies on many levels, that is, local, state, and national government and nongovernment entities that enforce health care requirements. This can frequently lead to many junctures at which differing requirements must be resolved.

This book has goals of sorting out the many ingredients necessary to build a health care facility and presenting them in such a way that the whole process can be appreciated and comprehended and showing how the multitude of requirements necessary in building or renovating a health care facility can be satisfied even when they differ in criteria.

Material for this book has been organized as much as possible in the order in which events occur. However, in the beginning stages of a project, several activities will almost assuredly have to take place simultaneously in order to make viable decisions. Individual circumstances will affect when and what needs to take place at any given moment. What is important, though, is that the governing body be cognizant of all the factors involved in the total project.

This book was written to provide assistance for all types of health care facility construction projects and for all types of persons involved in planning such projects or studying the process of building such facilities.

Types of projects include new construction of, additions to, or renovations to such facilities as hospitals (medical, rehabilitation, mental care), skilled nursing facilities, ambulatory health care centers, clinics, medical and dental offices, alcoholic rehabilitation centers, nursing homes, extended care facilities, residential custodial care facilities, and supervisory care facilities. It can also apply to parking garages, incinerators, medical office buildings, or satellite clinics that a health care facility needs to build. This book can also be useful for the newest types of facilities being built: the "medical-mall complex," where related retail shops, such as a pharmacy, medical equipment supplier, fitness center, and gift shop, are included in the complex; and convenience clinics that are being built as part of a retail mall or as malls unto themselves. (The latter, while not classified as health care occupancies, still have to consider many of the issues that health care facilities face, such as appropriate emergency electric power, handicapped accessibility, and radiation protection.) If what is to be built will be part of a health care facility, then this book's content is applicable. (As may be evident, there will be major differences in the work required to renovate a floor of a small hospital, as compared to the building of a large urban, multifunction medical center or the addition of a wing onto a nursing home.)

The individuals that this book addresses include administrators or chief executive officers of a facility and their staff; health care facility board members; building committees; medical facility plant engineers; enforcing authorities, both voluntary and regulatory; health care architects, designers, and engineers; contractors; financial advisers; business, economics, architecture, and engineering students who plan to enter the health care field; and medical and nursing personnel who are responsible for, or involved in, the building of a health care facility.

Why build a health care facility? It could be the result of a growing population; an aged building becoming too aged; or a desire of benefactors to help others by contributing to the building of a medical facility in honor or memory of someone. Whatever the reason, the result is a decision by some group, administration, or agency to build a particular type of health care facility in a certain location. Yet even that decision (or desire) cannot be considered final, as Part I of this book will show. Many hurdles must be successfully cleared before one spade of dirt can be overturned.

If someone does want to build a health care facility, why has it become so complex and at times downright frustrating? Why have so many constraints been imposed on the process of erecting facilities whose raison d'être will be the caring of the sick, the aged, and the handicapped? Part of the answer lies in the very type of activity to take place within such facilities: healing or caring for those who need professional assistance. Today, that healing or caring process can have patients deliberately unconscious for periods of time; it can involve restraining patients physically or by sedative-type medications; it can mean caring for infants who have absolutely no control over their actions in any situation; or it can involve patients of all ages who may not be able to comprehend even simple directions. Because the occupants of a health care facility will, in many instances, be partially or totally incapable of moving, being moved, or taking any measures of self-defense in an emergency, there is much concern that extra safety measures above the normal level be added to the design of these facilities. In fact, because of this situation, a philosophy of defend in place has evolved with respect to fire and the design of health care facilities: rather than the usual immediate exiting in an emergency, compartmentation (which creates areas of refuge) is designed into the structure so that minimal movement will be necessary.

Of course, health care facilities are not totally unique in their building requirements. As much as 80 percent of the construction parameters (e.g., columns, floors, walls, heating system, water and sewage system) are essentially the same as for other structures. They must meet the same criteria of adequate load-bearing capability, reasonable heating and cooling, removal of waste products, and other construction factors. However, it is the other 20 percent of construction that is different because of what takes place in a health care facility. These factors mean that additional or different construction measures need to be taken.

Even after construction, the operation of a health care facility requires more surveillance because of the nature of its activities and its special occupants. Any modifications, therefore, must be viewed with more than normal concern.

So the process of building a health care facility has become a complicated one. There are building codes, fire codes, health codes, inspection agencies, certificates of need, certifications, licensure, accreditation—all in order to build something to treat people. It is not easy, but it can be a very rewarding experience.

As we progress with further details on how a facility gets built, readers should remember that some portions of activities discussed in Part II can be conducted, and should be in some cases, during activities addressed in Part I. The sequencing of chapters in this book by no means matches that of events as might occur for all projects. Every project has unique features that will affect the order of activities. Although the material in this book covers the entire process of building or remodeling, the order of topics presented is a general one and should be adjusted for a particular project.

What follows is aimed at understanding that process in order to successfully build a safe and efficient health care facility.

We hope the material in this book will heighten awareness of what is involved in building a health care facility and of how the different parts of a project relate to each other. Building or renovating a health care facility should not be viewed as an insurmountable project. We thus hope this book will be useful reference source for both newcomers and seasoned veterans.

Have we included everything there is to know about building or renovating a health care facility? We would be kidding ourselves and the readers to even suggest it. However, we do feel we have placed under one cover a lot of material that heretofore was scattered throughout various books, documents, and articles. We also feel that it is the most comprehensive treatment of this subject to date. But since it is also the first of its kind, reader comments are most welcome.

Acknowledgments

We wish to thank Pat Boylan and Kathleen Montana for their assistance in typing portions of this book.

We also wish to thank The Ritchie Organization for the use of photographs that illustrate the process of building a health care facility. Also, a special thanks to the late James H. Ritchie, founder of The Ritchie Organization.

This book represents the cumulative knowledge and experience gained from many years of working with hundreds of persons involved in both the construction and operation of health care facilities. To name a few would be unkind to the many not named. But this book could not have been written if their paths in life had not crossed ours.

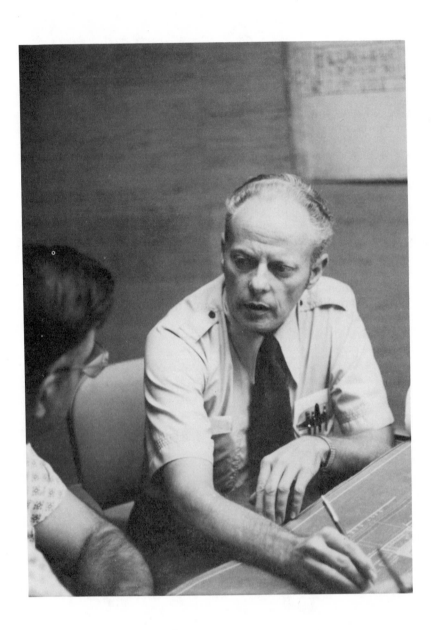

Part I

From 'An' Idea to 'The' Idea

CHAPTER 1

Defining What Is to Be Built

AN IDEA

So you want to build a health care facility. You are an administrator of a hospital or nursing home. Or you are a health care facility engineer or financial consultant. Or a member of the board of governors of a facility. Or a member of a building committee. Or an architect or an engineer. Or an insurance risk assessor. Or a city building inspector. Do you know what's involved — *all* that's involved?

Statistically, most persons within health care facilities have been involved in building a facility very few times. Consider how many times the average hospital adds a new wing. Every 10 to 20 years? Only a few individuals have participated in such projects many times. For most persons, then, knowing how all the pieces fit together and how they themselves fit into the total picture should be of concern. For it is the layperson's ability to convey the right information at the right time that enables the professional person to do his or her job and to produce a structure that reflects the needs of those who will have to work in it.

Balancing needs, desires, costs, and regulations in the construction of a new health care facility, an addition, or a major renovation of an existing health care facility requires knowledge of a host of complicated and interrelated activities. These include finance, economics, medical practices, enforcement requirements, and even public relations, to name a few. (Many of these activities are discussed in this book.) A person's ability to work under the constraints imposed on health care facilities today is directly related to his or her ability to know how to make the necessary activities happen, and happen at the right time.

3

Where does one find all there is to know about building a health care facility? Is there a cookbook for building a health care facility? No, and none is possible since there are no national codes that are all-inclusive. The documents of the National Fire Protection Association cover fire, electrical, and life safety; the Model Building Codes cover building aspects; each state has its own health requirements. This book serves as an introduction to all the activities or actions that are necessary in building a health care facility. Although every project is unique in some way, the contents of this book are applicable to all projects.

DEFINING THE PROJECT

In defining what it is to be built, one needs to consider and thoroughly analyze five questions, documenting answers for each. These questions are why? what? how? where? and when? Answering these five questions can be likened to the traditional feasibility study.

Why?

Why does something have to be built or renovated? What is the need? Is the plant in need of modernization because its efficiency has become unacceptable? Has the size of the present facility been stretched as far as it can? Are new activities not possible because of the existing facility's size? Or is enlargement of current activities not possible because there is not any more extra room or nothing can be reduced? Does the hospital or nursing home need or want more beds because occupancy rates are projected to increase? Has a nearby health care facility closed or reduced its capacity or services? Is the medical staff the impetus for some changes, that is, they want more space, but there isn't any in the existing structure? All these questions prod the question of Why is it necessary to build? The answers will be closely scrutinized by various groups, such as the Certificate of Need boards and local residents. (This is explained further in Chapter 2.)

What?

After answering satisfactorily to oneself why building is necessary, the next question that should be answered is, What should be built? The four major points here are type, size, function, and style.

- Type refers to the basic structure envisioned: a new hospital, a new nursing home, additional clinics, a new patient wing.

- Size depends on the functions and their number being proposed for the new structure: for example, a suite of operating rooms; general patient care areas; minor examination rooms. Size is the result of the cumulative addition of space required for each and all functions.

- Function refers to the activities that will take place in the new structure, such as surgery, nursing, business; psychiatry, diagnostics, laboratory testing. However, it is also subject to what the authorities allow to be built. (This is discussed in Chapter 3.) These new functions must also be analyzed in terms of how they relate to any existing functions.

- The style of the new structure describes the facade of the structure. It may be postmodern or colonial; brick, block, or wood. Sometimes there are external constraints on style, as in codes restricting what can be used. Sometimes there are existing constraints—for example, a new wing with respect to the existing building or a new structure with respect to an adjacent structure. Style may be constrained by location in the country, such as northern New England as opposed to the Southwest. Style can even be the result of the staff's preferences.

How?

This question requires a hard look at two distinct areas: operation and finance. The answers differ according to whether an organization is looking at building a new, separate structure or adding onto an existing structure. For a new structure, the major factor is money—that is, initial capital in order to build since there will be no income until services are started. (This subject of finance is discussed in detail in Chapter 3.) With respect to adding to an existing structure, concern is for maintaining services; otherwise, as with any other company, the customer (i.e., the patient) will go elsewhere. Health care delivery is very competitive today.

Where?

This may appear to have a simple answer, but determining the location of the structure can be just as complicated as answering the three previous questions. The term *location* refers not to the design location of the new addition or new structure but rather to the geographic location. And the best or right location may not always be possible, as discussed later in this section and also in Chapter 5, in which the subject of land is covered. Many factors, including internal ones if the new structure is an addition to an existing structure, affect the final location.

If the new structure is to be an addition to an existing structure, the location is obvious: tangential to some portion of an existing wall. Thus the best tangential point has to be decided. If the new structure is to be a separate, freestanding structure, the location is more complicated to determine and may involve many additional factors.

The following factors influence the final location of a new structure. Although some apply to both an addition and a separate new structure, others apply to just one or the other. Each needs to be reviewed for its effect on a particular project.

External. External factors include the following:

1. Environmental considerations (e.g., hills, rocks, rivers, water table, soil, substrata). These weigh heavily on any structure and are discussed in detail in Chapter 5.

2. Traffic and access. Local regulations on street parking need to be studied; jurisdictional questions may have to be answered with respect to local, state, and even federal road access.

3. Location of nearest fire departments, their response times, and the ready accessibility of all portions of the facility by fire department apparatus and personnel after the new structure is completed.

4. Location of other medical services that may be needed (e.g., a nursing home in relation to a hospital).

5. Transfer capabilities of police, fire, and ambulance services in case of a disaster (either internal or external disaster) and sites that can be utilized for such transfers.

6. Utility capabilities, such as electricity, water, gas, and sewage. Their location and access can affect where the facility can be located. (This is discussed further in Chapter 4.)

7. Public transportation. The availability of this service can have a significant influence.

8. Parking. This is always a major item, presenting one of the biggest problems and challenges. Adequate parking may take up more space than is available or than can be given up from other portions of the project. A parking garage is always a possible solution. A total parking review should include staff, patient, visitor, and emergency medical vehicle needs.

Internal. For existing facilities, where activities are currently being conducted within a facility also must be considered since they are, and will be, related to the new wing or structure. As an example, should all of radiology services be moved to the new wing, or should only pediatric radiology be moved if the new wing will be only pediatric? Or, if radiology services are located adjacent to where the wing is being considered, is enlargement better for handling the new pediatric wing rather than having two separate operations? Thus, disruption of services needs to be considered when locating the addition. Also, the overall flow of people and goods must be reviewed (for both staff and patients) to determine optimum efficiency of both.

When?

When to build or modify a health care facility depends on several seemingly unrelated factors. The following is a list of the more common ones.

- When any restrictions on the Certificate of Need have been met or cleared
- When the weather is appropriate (such as springtime so that concrete can be poured, or before winter so that framing will be enclosed)
- When community concerns have been met
- When completion of the project is desired
- When finances are in order

"When" is a two-edged proposition—balancing how well an owner or institution can complete what is needed against how soon the project is needed by a community.

CONCLUSION

The remaining chapters in Part I will explore these five questions in greater detail. But it is stressed again that many portions of Part I must be determined concurrently, since Part I is about determining the feasibility of erecting a building, i.e., are there any restrictions financially, physically, or legally? These three facets are very much interrelated. Hence, it becomes necessary to look at all three as one package and at the same time.

It is also very probable that some money will have to be spent in order to find out the answers to these questions. Facility owners or administrators should be aware that, even after spending this money, they may not be able to build what they want. It is thus a good practice to address the most formidable obstacles first, so that the least amount of money will have been spent if it turns out that the project cannot be completed.

Finally, it is necessary that the steps in Part I be accomplished and authorization received before much, if any, effort and money are expended working on the activities in Part II of this book: The Design Stage.

CHAPTER 2

Certificate of Need

Although the owners or operators of a health care facility may firmly believe that they need to build a new facility or add to an existing one, others may disagree. Some of these others may in fact have the authority to prevent the project from going forward. One such group is a board called the Certificate of Need (CON) board. These boards are rather autonomous in their responsibilities and authorities. What and who these boards are, and how they came to have such far-ranging authority, is the subject of this chapter.

HISTORY

In order to understand CON boards, one must know some history surrounding them. The major point to keep in mind is the intent of the federal and state governments, now and in the past, to try to keep the cost of medical care within the economic reach of all citizens. CON boards were just one manifestation of many efforts in this regard.

Advancements in medical practice have occurred sporadically but continuously over the years. These include the introduction of anesthesia in the 1860s, the use of electrical devices from the 1920s, and the transfusion of blood from the 1930s. Each event, however, had an interesting side effect: in addition to curing or alleviating a problem, it allowed physicians to treat even more patients and more serious problems. But since people don't buy health care the same way they buy cars or refrigerators (i.e., one can decide to forgo buying a car one year, or buy two the next; one cannot ignore a broken neck, high fever, or chest pains), the advancement in medicine, particularly during and immediately following World War II, placed strains and incentives on health care administrators. For a variety of reasons, the end result was a dramatically increasing cost to treat patients, even those with minor ailments. This increase was particularly noticeable in the area of construction.

In an attempt to help hospitals that felt the need and/or pressure to expand and control costs through such assistance, Congress passed the Hospital Survey and Construction Act in 1946. It came to be popularly known as the Hill-Burton Act (named after the two sponsors of the act). The act did several things. It authorized grants to states to survey health care facilities' needs of communities and establish adequate hospitals, clinics, and other facilities for all people. (In 1954, the act was amended to include public and voluntary nonprofit nursing homes.) It also required each state to designate a single state agency and advisory council to implement a program and establish a plan for surveying existing health care facilities in order to develop a program for needed construction.

Thus began direct federal and state government involvement in the decision process involving the construction of new health care facilities. (This later extended to all capital expenditures exceeding a certain value: originally more than $100,000.[1]) States for their part created agencies, or added staff to existing agencies, to fulfill federal requirements in order to obtain funds. According to a 1978 publication of the then health division of the U.S. Department of Health, Education, and Welfare (now the Department of Health and Human Services), states began enacting CON laws as early as 1964.[2] According to a recent Department of Health and Human Services publication,[3] 46 states and three territories now have CON programs, though about half do not comply with federal requirements (e.g., have less stringent requirements than federal requirements). These state CON laws continued to vary even after October 1972, when Congress passed P.L. 92-603 and amended the Social Security Act. Among other things, this act reinforced CON institutions by states and made clear the role of the federal government in not supporting unnecessary capital expenditures. The leverage for this latter item was in the form of the control of reimbursement funds (such as through Medicare). Although Section 1122 of P.L. 92-603 required a formal agreement between state and federal governments, it remained voluntary for states to enter into an agreement. However, Congress passed another act in 1974, P.L. 93-641, the National Health Planning and Resources Development Act. This act required states to develop and administer CON programs through state health system agencies. Although CON programs vary for political and economic reasons, generally they were established to review the state's health care delivery needs and determine if a particular project was within the objectives or guidelines established.

CON BOARDS AND MEMBERS

With P.L. 92-603 and 93-641, states were required to establish, if they had not already, legally empowered government agencies to make a determination of need of projects and issue, when the project is approved, a certificate approving the expenditure. Whatever mechanism is established in the state bureaucracy, the group that performs the first review is the local CON board (see next section).

Members of CON boards are selected from a cross section of the public, with a state agency (e.g., department of public health) providing administrative support, such as meeting rooms, correspondence, and documentation. The number of board members ranges from 6 to 12, with alternates in some instances. Representatives include, but are not limited to, physicians, nurses, retail merchants, lawyers, and the general consumer. Only one representative from each sector is allowed on a board. The intent is that the board should represent a cross section of the economy.

Board positions are not full-time, and no terms of office are called for, though states may establish them. Appointment to boards can be made by the governor, lieutenant governor, or commissioner of public health. Some states provide partial reimbursement (e.g., travel expenses), but generally board members serve on a voluntary basis.

Because membership on a board is by appointment, there is considerable lobbying, as might be expected, as to who is selected.

ACTIVITIES OF CON BOARDS
AND HEALTH CARE FACILITIES

During this definition stage, health care facility owners or administrators must submit letters of intent to their local CON board. This means the facility must know *whom* to contact, *when* to contact, and *what* to submit. The "who" can be ascertained through relatively few telephone calls. The "when" and "what" require more work. Letters of intent must contain details concerning all five questions discussed in Chapter 1 (i.e., why facility wants something built; what is desired to be built; how the facility expects to build it; where the structure is to be built; and when is facility to be built). Thus, when letters of intent should be submitted depends on when these answers are known. Professional judgment is obviously needed. Submissions may be very detailed or very general in concept and planning or any combination thereof.

The CON board, in fulfilling its responsibilities, reviews each submission and then takes one of the following actions: it can approve the project as submitted; it can specify the total cost that can be spent; or it can even tell the facility what it (the board) feels the facility should build or needs to build. Almost without exception, CON boards downgrade the extent of projects. CON boards can even tell owners or operators of the facility how much time they have to build the desired structure or renovate the existing one. Approval to build is not open-ended regarding time (see also the section And Also a Plan to Spend Money in Chapter 3).

What do CON boards base their decisions on? Current services and future utilization. The board reviews services currently available from existing health care facilities in the area and how well, or to what extent, they are being utilized. As an example, if a hospital wanted to add 100 beds, a CON board would take into consideration the bed census of nearby facilities as part of its review.

CON boards do vary in the extent of their duties. Some review health care activities within a certain radius (e.g., 10 miles, 50 miles); others have authority within the same local political subdivision or within one county or within the entire state. Boards are relatively free to base their judgments on whatever they deem appropriate. A health care facility thus needs to know whether it will be duplicating existing services or creating new ones. If it will be doing the former, it must be able to document and describe why additional services are needed. If it will be providing new services, its plans are less likely to be disapproved by the CON board.

One interesting aspect of the CON process is the public review a project is given or subjected to. This is to assess the societal impact of a new or additional health care facility. Thus, area residents should be apprised by owners of their intentions early in this process, highlighting the benefits of the project. The temporary inconveniences of noise, dirt, and other construction annoyances should not be ignored, however. Rather, the methods that will be used to minimize these inconveniences should be stressed.

Finally, the CON process involves local CON boards sending their recommendations on a project to a state agency (e.g., a health systems agency or a state health planning and development agency). The state-level agency will review the CON board recommendations, either approve or modify them, and then forward the entire matter to the federal government (U.S. Department of Health and Human Services) for final approval. Outright rejection by Health and Human Services has been very rare.

If and when all agencies, both state and federal, approve a project, CON boards send the owners a form (EC-4) stating what has been approved and for how long approval of the project is valid and requiring that the owners build or renovate the facility as proposed or approved by the CON board. This form must be signed and returned to the CON board. During construction, another CON form (EC-8) is sent to owners, asking whether the project is being built per the approved plans and whether proposed expenditures are being exceeded. This form also must be signed and returned to the CON board.

As may be evident, the activities of a CON board extend beyond the initial approval of a project.

TRENDS

With a change in federal government policy relative to health care reimbursement for Medicare and Medicaid patients, the role of CON boards in the construction of health care facilities may also change. Because Medicare and Medicaid patients represent a significant percentage of patients today, the need for and effectiveness of CON boards in controlling health care costs may diminish. The original purpose of CON boards (to control "bed construction") may have run its course after 20 years. Although CON boards are heavily controlled at the state level, funds for construction originate in many instances at the federal level. If this source dries up, much of current CON boards' purposes will be affected.

As a result, from a construction and economics perspective, the normal supply and demand operative might return as the major factor in determining the amount of construction. In lieu of CON boards, the federal government may control construction through tighter control on reimbursements.

Complicating and affecting all of the above is the interesting paradox that the inflation rate has dropped substantially in the past few years, yet patient costs are continuing to rise. If construction is left to seek its own equilibrium, CON boards will have to concentrate more of their efforts to control costs through other factors, such as labor costs.

If trends do not shift and the cost of medical care continues to rise as fast as it has in the recent past (with the result that it becomes more and more unaffordable), the heavy hand of the federal government will most likely be forced to act on behalf of its citizenry. Health care delivery will not be allowed to become a privilege of a few. And CON boards will be affected by whatever changes are made.

NOTES

1. A note of caution: It is not worth trying to circumvent the CON process, such as by dividing a $1 million project into two $500,000 projects. Although attempts to do so are made all the time, the CON process is too thorough to attempt such subterfuge. A proposal that presents all the facts and costs up front is more apt to find a positive response, as opposed to a proposal that has some sudden unexpected costs after initial review.

2. *Certificate of Need Programs: A Review, Analysis and Annotated Bibliography of the Research Literature* (see Bibliography).

3. *Status Report on State Certificate of Need Programs* (see Bibliography).

CHAPTER 3

Financing

Building a health care facility is a costly endeavor. In fact, one of the major questions a Certificate of Need (CON) board asks a submitter of a project is how the money to complete the project will be obtained. A CON board generally requests a financial statement of how money will be secured.

Money to finance a project can be obtained from several sources: conventional borrowing via a mortgage, issuance of stocks or bonds, fund-raising, and grants. The first two methods are similar in that both require a repayment of the principal amount plus interest.

Each state has financing laws concerning how money can be secured for erecting a structure. These laws differ from state to state, so they need to be reviewed carefully and individually.

A financial consultant should be retained to assist and determine the best method of obtaining funds for the particular project. (See Chapter 7 for a discussion of financial consultants.) Financing and taxes are inseparable. If large amounts of money will be generated, a financial expert must examine state and federal tax laws to ensure that taxes do not reduce that amount generated before construction even begins.

THE MOST EXPENSIVE WAY

Borrowing money is the most expensive way of obtaining money since the interest rate charged must be higher than anything the lender can receive through investment elsewhere. Since financing laws vary from state to state, financial options regarding bank loans must be reviewed. Although banking regulations can appear to make all banks seem equal, regulations do allow some room for negotiation. Thus, shopping for the best deal is not restricted to buying a car. It includes securing a loan to build a health care facility. A fraction of a percentage point can mean a large difference in the total amount repaid, even if the project is a small addition to an existing facility.

The search for borrowing money should not be limited geographically. Since the economies vary from state to state, the availability of money to borrow can differ. Banks in other areas may be eager to expand or diversify their operations; those in an expansive phase may be more willing to negotiate than those in a consolidating phase. The services of a financial consultant (Chapter 7) may be useful in the long term in obtaining the best rate and/or the least extras (e.g., pay-back time, surcharges, points).

The search for lenders is not and should not be limited to banks. The federal government, through such agencies as the Departments of Health and Human Services and Housing and Urban Development, provides loans if the institution is, or will be, accredited for Medicare/Medicaid reimbursement. The advantage is that the federal government insures that the money is repaid. There are restrictions, of course, as to what the government will insure, for example, nonprofit facilities only.

THE STOCKS AND BONDS WAY

A less expensive way of obtaining funds is through the issuance of stocks or bonds. Again, each state has its own laws as to how a private institution can issue such instruments. The advantage of the bond method over a mortgage is that the facility becomes a sort of bank, with a lower rate of interest having to be paid than for borrowing the same amount from a bank. Bonds issued by a health care facility are like U.S. Savings Bonds: for a set amount, the facility agrees to return the invested amount with interest after a predetermined time. Thus, instead of a facility obtaining money from financial institutions, it becomes its own financial institution, attracting depositors in the form of bondholders. In some states, a nonprofit health care facility can issue tax-free bonds to bondholders.

Funding through the issuance of stock offerings has even more financial advantages for a facility than using the bond method: financial risks are shared among those who purchase stock. Should the facility not generate projected revenues as expected or in the time estimated, the value of the stock will reflect it and the amount a facility has to repay when a share of stock is redeemed will be correspondingly lower. However, financial rewards are also shared by those who purchase stock. Higher profits can increase the value of the stock or can be shared with stockholders through higher dividends. The facility does not lose money; its profits are just less since stockholders share in the increased value of the stock. In both instances, through the sharing of financial obligations, a facility's financial exposure is lowered, both on the front end (i.e., raising money) and the back end (i.e., repaying money).

These first two methods of acquiring money do involve the dimension of repayment: the facility has to recover the amount borrowed and repay the lender or bondholder or stockholder the original amount plus interest or a dividend. This repayment may be in monthly, quarterly, or semiannual installments. To recover the amount borrowed, the facility must generate revenue. Revenue can be generated in the following ways:[1]

1. Charge patients for medical services rendered

2. Conduct research for a fee

3. Receive rental income on property owned

4. Initiate group services (e.g., laboratory, clinic, or walk-in facilities) to accommodate several hospitals, nursing homes, or other facilities

5. Request donations (see subsequent section, Donations) by conducting a fund-raising campaign or seeking contributions through wills and trusts

6. Establish a gift shop or coffee shop activity within the facility

7. Charge for parking

8. Apply for private, state, or federal grants (see subsequent section, The Grants Way)

9. Allow certain portions of the new facility or area to be "purchased" through a donation, with a suitable plaque of acknowledgment (e.g., This room possible through the generous support of the John B. Smith family.)

DONATIONS

Fund-raising is serious business. Raising money this way means selling something without directly giving something in return, except a grateful thank you or some token of appreciation. Fund-raising means convincing people that it is worth their while to help build a new wing or building. With so many other groups and organizations making similar solicitations for their work or projects, raising money in this manner must be done thoughtfully and seriously. Today, there are firms that specialize in fund-raising.

Some persons may be convinced, or voluntarily decide, to donate money through bequeathals. For the final amount transferred to be maximized, the inheritance laws of the state where the person resided and the state in which the facility is located or incorporated (if different) should be reviewed.

A variation on donations is the use of lotteries. Here, significant amounts of money are given away as an inducement to attract a large number of persons to buy low-priced tickets. Because this method is a form of gambling, a review of state lottery regulations is a prerequisite to establishing a lottery. Also, staff, board members, local volunteer groups, and others should be consulted to determine if this method is considered offensive to their staff, members, or local citizenry.

THE GRANTS WAY

The fourth way of obtaining money might be considered a form of fund-raising: obtaining a grant. In this case, some organization or agency actually has money that it wants to give away just for the asking. However, there are usually conditions that must be met in order to receive such money (e.g., raising matching funds; conducting research in a specific area). Whatever the reason for the giveaway, all that is usually required is a detailed application explaining how much money is desired, why it is needed, and who will benefit as a result. There will also have to be written (legal) assurance that money so granted will be spent as requested.

Following written applications, personal interviews and even site visits may be conducted by the grantor. These last two activities are usually dependent on the amount of money being granted.

After a grant is awarded, periodic reports may have to be submitted, and additional progress visits by a representative of the grantor might be required.[2] After the project is completed, a final report may even be requested.

Thus, although a grant may seem like a donation since there is no direct repayment, it is a regulated donation that can be revoked if the money is not spent in the way originally intended. This is not to say that some grants are very general in stating what can be done with the award and others are so specific that it is relatively easy to meet the terms of the award. However, grants generally have a certain amount of oversight attached to them. Owners should thus become cognizant of it and not run the risk of losing the award.

Whatever method or methods of raising money are used, the total required should first be determined. The amount to be raised should equal (and, for contingency purposes, slightly exceed) the amount needed so that obligations can be met. In addition, contingency plans should be developed in the event that original fund-raising efforts fall short of target (e.g., expected grants are not awarded; the economy or donations in the area turn downward; bequeathers change their minds while still possible). A financial committee should thus be formed and a financial consultant retained to manage the acquisitions, investment, and expenditure of money raised. (See Chapter 7 on selecting a financial consultant.)

AND ALSO A PLAN TO SPEND MONEY

On the other side of the financial coin is the plan for spending money in order to build and operate the new wing or structure. CON boards (see Chapter 2) like to be assured that an existing facility will be able to not only build a new facility but also operate it. Thus, the following information must be submitted to the CON board:

1. A proposed overall operating budget for the next 3 to 5 years, based on the assumption that the new wing or structure is completed on time. This should include a proposed rate schedule that is within the reach of the population to be served.

2. A statement of why the proposed plan has at least one more advantage than other possible plans, such as building a new

wing as opposed to a separate structure. Advantages should be stated in terms of initial cost, long-term costs, and patient-cost benefit, indicating any reduction in patient costs because of the new facility.

3. A description of the construction method to be used (i.e., the least costly method without compromising quality or safety)

4. A summary of how construction costs will be managed. This includes:

- Actual construction and building costs, including major equipment such as kitchen equipment, X-ray units, heating units

- Cost of furniture and movable equipment

- Site costs, such as surveys, borings, and the meeting of environmental impact requirements (see Chapter 5)

- Architectural, engineering, and consultant fees

- Fund-raiser fees

- Legal fees

- Noncontractor construction costs (e.g., clerk of the works fees, utilities, insurance, and contingency funding)

ASSETS

Holdings include property, interest in buildings (e.g., a doctor's office building), trusts, and stock portfolios. All holdings must be disclosed since they affect a facility's income. Because records are scrutinized by CON boards, a complete accounting should be prepared. This matter can be very complex if a facility has diversified holdings. The retention of a financial consultant may be worth much more than the cost of the consultant.

ESTIMATING COSTS

One final point related to financing is estimating the cost of building the new structure. Although final, firm figures are not possible at this stage, rough estimates are possible and necessary. Revealing the approximate cost of the venture when going before CON boards, prospective investors, or donors will show that an owner is serious as well as knowledgeable. Owners can receive assistance from professional cost estimators.

NOTES

1. A facility could also deposit in the bank some or most of the money it borrows or receives but does not need initially (such as in certificates of deposits or other high-yield instruments). It is rare that all the money received through loans, grants, or other means will have to be spent initially. The interest received will thus help reduce the actual cost of the original loan or the amount that has to be repaid to investors.

2. Appropriate recognition of large grants should be included in press releases, ground-breaking ceremonies, dedication ceremonies, and so on (see Chapters 13 and 16).

CHAPTER 4

Zoning Restrictions and Code Implications

Through zoning, cities and towns prevent random erection of structures within their jurisdiction and control what is erected.

WHY ZONING?

Zoning means more than setting the boundaries of lots within a city or town. The size of lots, established through zoning, affects the size of the structure that can be placed on the lot. Height restrictions (or limitations), also established through zoning, affect the type of structure that can be erected.

Factors affecting zoning include utility capabilities; desired densities; aesthetics; even history (i.e., what structures already exist in the area, their size, their height, and how long they have been there can have a bearing). Once an area is zoned, it does not mean that the area cannot be rezoned or that deviations from established rules for that zone will not be allowed (e.g., allowance for a taller structure than the area is zoned for or changing the dimensions of two adjacent lots to accommodate the special needs in one of the lots).

One typical situation is a community hospital wanting to build in an area zoned for residential use only. For the benefit of the persons who will need its services, many hospitals try to locate their facilities near the residents they will be serving. As a result, hospital administrations must go before local zoning boards and present arguments as to why the board should grant a waiver to the rules for that zone. This procedure is necessary not only initially but also whenever a hospital wants to erect additions to its building(s).

Utilities such as communications, water (domestic and fire), sewage (domestic and storm), gas, electricity, and steam are related to zoning in the following way. When a zoning board classifies areas of a town or city for particular types of structures (e.g., residential one-family units; residential up-to-four units; residential hi-rise apartments; commercial one-story; commercial up-to-six stories), the utilities necessary to support the levels of activities expected can be estimated rather closely. Once areas are zoned, sewer lines, electrical power cables, telephone cables, and other equipment can be roughed in or even partially installed. However, if the zoning board reclassifies an area as one that will allow more persons or increased activities, additional or larger sewer lines may be necessary, additional power and telephone lines will have to be installed, and so on. Thus, any changes in the zoning of an area that already has structures within it or is partially developed must consider the effect of a change in zoning on the utilities available or planned for that area.

A relatively new factor required by zoning boards is the inclusion of adequate parking facilities for staff, patients, visitors, and handicapped. For handicapped parking, zoning boards even direct how many spaces are to be provided. In addition, parking requirements extend to proper lighting, sidewalk access, drainage, and even snow removal. For this last item, there may have to be sufficient land surrounding the parking area to pile the snow. Otherwise, parking spaces would be reduced by the presence of snow.

Most communities today are concerned about what is being built within their boundaries, particularly from property value and environmental points of view. As a result, in conjunction with some zoning boards, land use committees now review proposed buildings. These committees take a more esoteric view than zoning boards of the land within the boundaries of a city or town and review such issues as population density and the city or town's present and future building character.

RELATIONSHIP OF CODES TO ZONING

Zoning and codes can be considered together since they are related: both set up criteria (restrictions) as to what can take place or be built. For that reason, at the local level, the city or town building commissioner or inspector usually is involved in zoning activities.

As to which parameter should be looked at first, zoning considerations take priority. Can one build a proposed structure in a particular location? Does the new structure meet the zoning criteria of the zone where it is to be erected?

A health care facilities owner must first show a zoning board that the land in question is clear from encumbrances, such as rights of ways, restricted heights, and set backs. It must then, if necessary, submit petitions for any variances it seeks to the requirements for that zoned area.

After the zoning hurdle is cleared, the effect of codes can be judged.[1] Here the question concerns the level of building. For example, can a one-story nursing home be constructed of wood, or must it be made of a fire-resistant material? Does a multistory structure have sufficient fire service access?

Another zoning and code implication factor that health care facilities should be aware of is the type of building that is possible. This is based on fire safety purposes as well as on building construction purposes. Thus, if a height of 100 feet is allowed, NFPA 220,[2] Standard on Types of Building Construction, and NFPA 101, Life Safety Code, outline the type of building possible based on material and the presence of a sprinkler system. The building codes, however, define such a building based on structural considerations. As might be expected, there is some overlap between fire safety and building codes. If differences between the two do exist, they must be reconciled.

NOTES

1. The codes referred to here relate to zoning. In Chapter 11, codes relating to construction are discussed.

2. Throughout this book, NFPA refers to the National Fire Protection Association.

CHAPTER 5

The Land (Above, On, Below)

A structure is able to exist because of what is below the ground, on the land, and even above the land. This may seem like a simplistic statement, but in fact these factors are a very complicated prerequisite for building any structure. Information about the land must be known before the piece of land can be considered acceptable for a new structure.

Complicating the factors further is the issue of knowing what type of structure is desired, its configuration, its structural features, and its anticipated loads. For example, will it be a one-story building or a twenty-story building? A 20-by-50-foot building or a 200-by-300-foot building? A building with no basement, a regular basement, or a subbasement? A building with average loads or one with a 50-ton device on the third floor?

In this chapter, the influence of the land surrounding the structure is discussed. Once this information is known, the latitude in building extent can be determined.

Factors that affect the selection of a particular parcel of land can be grouped as follows:

1. Environmental (both natural and imposed)

2. Geological configuration and activities

3. Foundation prerequisites

4. Societal influences

It should be remembered that these factors are considerably interrelated and thus require simultaneous review when making a decision on the land.

ENVIRONMENTAL

Nature has first dibs on what can be built anywhere on this earth. Governments are finally realizing this and are instituting regulations more in harmony with nature to help retain the fundamental balance of nature that existed before humans started erecting structures. The recent serious building boom has wrought havoc with what is a very delicate balance.

What are some of the natural environmental conditions that can affect the building of a structure, particularly a health care facility, in an area? The *terrain* of the land is one. Sides of hills can be beautiful to see from or be seen from, but they can be formidable for patients, the handicapped, and the elderly to negotiate. Although ramps, escalators, and elevators can offset this problem, they can add much cost to a project. They also add an extra burden for fire departments and evacuation teams should movement from the building be necessary. Winter conditions in some parts of the country also make access difficult for patients, who are not always ambulatory. Thus, terrain as level as possible for as much time as possible is desirable.

Wind is refreshing if moderate but treacherous if too heavy. Thus, a relatively new consideration when building a structure is knowing or estimating what type of wind conditions will be created around a structure. This is of particular concern to health care facilities, where the population of handicapped, elderly, and other physically challenged individuals will be more concentrated. These persons will not be as capable as others of buffeting themselves against strong winds.

Wind direction should also be considered. Is the site generally upwind or downwind from industries that emit unpleasant or unhealthy fumes or smoke? How close is the source of these problems?

In the Northwest, it is necessary to ask how close the nearest active volcano is since winds carry the products of an erupting volcano aloft and deposit them hundreds of miles downwind.

Water conditions, both above and below ground, need to be considered. Are there constant flood conditions when it rains, or have measures been taken to channel runoff, prevent soil erosion, and eliminate other potential damage. What has the water table been like over the past 25 years? Has it remained relatively stable, is it rising or is it dropping?

Although nature's surface and above-surface environmental

state is not static, human beings have done some very unkind things to upset a rather precious balance. In this regard, local, state, and federal agencies have been passing ordinances and regulations. Some of these are directed at the land and air to prevent further disruption to the balance. Others are directed at the type of buildings or activities that will be permitted in an area. These ordinances and regulations can, in turn, be incorporated into zoning laws or referenced by zoning boards (see Chapter 4). Environmental regulations should thus be investigated thoroughly.

Because natural weather conditions (e.g., rain, snow) cannot be changed, developers of hospitals, nursing homes, clinics, and other facilities will not have the luxury of negating all adverse conditions. However, the environment cannot be ignored when building a health care facility, particularly because the building will be housing persons who are not well.

GEOLOGICAL CONFIGURATION AND ACTIVITIES

How the earth is arranged below the surface and what, if anything, is going on down under are important factors in determining what can be built in an area. Test borings or sonic soundings are thus necessary to learn what exists 10 feet, 50 feet, or even 100 feet below the surface (depending on what structure is contemplated). Is there silt, sand, swamp, or water below, or is there a ridge of solid rock?

The other major geological concern is earth movement (i.e., tremors, quakes, faults). This has generally been of concern only in regions west of the Rocky Mountains, but such movements have occurred in other areas.

Subsoil data must be obtained from a professional involved in this field prior to any design work.

FOUNDATION PREREQUISITES

Although the geology of an area cannot be changed, some latitude exists with respect to the base (foundation) upon which a structure will sit. There are many types of foundation solutions, such as piles, floating foundations, and variations of common foundations. However, these types cost many dollars above those spent for a normal situation, and a thorough investigation must be made to determine if the extra cost is worth it.

Thus, geology and foundation must be known. Once the former is known, the possible types of foundation can be studied and calculations made based on the geology and weight or loads of the proposed structure.

Generally, providing environmental data is not the responsibility of the architect. The owner must learn what conditions prevail above the land, what controls have been instituted for the land, and what conditions exist below the land. Surveys of a parcel of land will have to be conducted by knowledgeable persons at the direction of owners. These surveys must include not only the topographical features of the surface but also the condition of the land below. Test borings, the digging of a trench, or sonic surveys may be necessary to learn what exists below the surface.

The architect or engineer can assist the owner in several ways, however. This includes locating where the work should be done and determining who are the proper professionals to do the work.

All information so gathered (the survey of the surface and the testing of the subsoil) must be thoroughly documented and recorded.

SOCIETAL INFLUENCES

In addition to considering natural conditions below the land and environmental conditions above the land, the owner must pay attention to the human condition related to the land since it will affect the location of the facility. Although natural factors cannot be changed except by relocating the structure, if possible, human factors can be altered, shifted, or changed because society is generally more flexible than nature.

Some of the more prominent societal influences as they affect the location of a health care facility include the following.

Vehicular Access and Expandability

Since a new or expanded facility creates more traffic, whether the surrounding area can accommodate these additional loads must be considered. The number and type of roads should be analyzed. A facility might have to share road-building expenses as a result.

Potential Patients

This is a marketing question: will there be a sufficient number of patients within the service area of the facility who will want to be able to utilize the proposed services of the facility? For proposed facilities that are considering the inclusion of surgical services, the question may extend to day surgery or walk-in medical care and whether this type of care will be offered.

Potential Staff

This is a more controllable factor than the previous one in that the quantity and type of staff needed are quantifiable. However, there have to be incentives to attract staff. Is the area pleasant as opposed to tolerable? Will salaries be competitive with those of other health care facilities in the area? Are there good schools and universities in the area? The study must include *all* persons to be hired (medical, nursing, technical, support, personnel, and administrative) who are necessary to operate a health care facility.

Competition

The delivery of medical services is a business. As such, many of the rules of business will apply. Are there other health care facilities offering the same services? Is there room for competition? Will a new facility enable group purchasing of supplies? Will there be incentives for people to use the new facility?

Societal influences indeed have an effect on the location of any new facility and thus need to be fully explored during the early phases of this process.

CHAPTER 6

Structural Considerations

This chapter is an extension of Chapters 4 and 5, in which zoning and the land were discussed. It addresses some of the structural factors that affect the type of structure that can be built.

The structure of a building is the basic skeleton upon which the entire facility is erected. A great deal of consideration must go into deciding which system is best for the particular project.

As an aid to the reader, factors will be divided into three categories: those common to both additions and new structures; those applicable just to additions to existing structures; and those applicable just to new structures. Following this, some details of various types of structures are discussed.

COMMON TO ANY STRUCTURE

Whether a project is an addition to an existing structure or a new structure, several considerations that are applicable to both can affect the type and extent of the structure that can be built. These include:

1. Subsoil level

2. Foundation

3. Proneness to earthquakes

4. Fire-resistive classification

5. Occupancy classification

6. Fireproofing requirements

7. Structural loading requirements

Subsoil Level

The status of the subsoil below the site of the proposed structure is most necessary because it determines how heavy (large) a structure can be erected on the site. In the case of an existing building, it cannot be assumed that the subsoil adjacent to the building will be satisfactory just because of this adjacency. New tests have to be conducted.

Foundation

The subsoil data must be obtained prior to any decision about the type of structure desired. Such items as rock, water, sand, swamp, gravel, and artificial fill will determine what type of foundation is possible and appropriate. For example, will caissons or piles be needed? Will a basement prove too risky because of water conditions? Will elevator pits need to be blasted out because of rock presence? The importance of obtaining subsoil information cannot be overstated. It will have a direct bearing on the cost of the structure because of its effect on the foundation that must be built. All good structures are built on firm foundations.

When discussions on foundations are held, the immediate plans as well as the long-range plans for the institution should be considered. Foundations that can handle future floors, as an example, will be well worth the investment.

Proneness to Earthquakes

If the area is within a known earthquake zone, appropriate measures must be taken for the new structure, particularly if it is adjacent to an existing building that may or may not have had earthquake measures built in.

Fire Rating

Fire and building codes specify what fire-resistive rating each type of structure is required to meet. This applies to wood-framed, steel, concrete structures, and any combination thereof. This specification or rating is in terms of the fire-resistive rating for the structural frame, walls, and floor and ceiling assemblies.

NFPA 220, Standard Types of Building Construction, defines the construction type of fire-resistive rating of building components. For example, a Type I (443) building has 4-hour fire-resistive-rated exterior load-bearing walls, 4-hour structural frame, and 3-hour floors.

NFPA 101, Life Safety Code, in turn states what building construction type is acceptable for a given occupancy in a given situation.

Occupancy Classification

Fire and building codes also place restrictions on the type of structure that can be built, based on the expected occupancy of the structure. A one-story addition to an existing nursing home will differ significantly from a new 15-story hospital. But local authorities can make the classification even more restricted.

Fireproofing Requirements

The extent of a new addition or structure will also dictate the amount of fireproofing necessary — whether protection can be sprayed on, what type of walls are allowed, and how many smoke barriers are necessary for each floor.[1]

Structural loading requirements

Finally, the type of activities to take place in the new addition or structure will affect the type of structure that can be built. Structural configuration will vary considerably between an auditorium, a library, a hydrotherapy room, a cobalt treatment room, and a row of patient rooms.

AN ADDITION

When the new structure is an addition to an existing structure, continuity is a major factor in deciding what will be built. How different can the exterior of the addition be without clashing with that of the existing structure? Although the interior framing does not need to be identical, careful consideration of the facing, windows, and doors must be made. Aesthetics can thus impact on the structural aspects of the building.

The desired location of the addition affects the type of structure that can be erected. A sloping open grade presents one situation; an abutting parking lot another. Whereas owners may want the new structure in one place, the land may present additional costs or sufficient obstacles to preclude the kind of structure desired or to shift its location to a less efficient one.

In addition to exterior factors, internal pass-throughs, changes in exiting requirements, and structural integrity at interface points must be considered.

Internal pass-throughs will be necessary at each level to connect the two structures and to provide means of exiting. The location of these pass-throughs should be as least disruptive as possible, such as by extending the natural flow of existing corridors. In this regard, the question of whether to have floor-to-floor heights the same as those of the existing structure and/or at the same horizontal level needs to be decided. Keeping these two factors the same will reduce differential structuring and permit the joining of pass-throughs.

Although the existing structure may provide exiting capability for the new structure, a new addition might also create exiting problems or interfere with exiting designs and evacuation plans of the exiting structure. Thus, the design of the new structure will have to take exiting requirements, in total, under consideration.

Structural integrity at interface points must take into consideration the age and design of the existing structure so that the new structure does not weaken the existing structure at interface points. This is particularly critical at pass-through points, where a large opening will be created in the wall of the existing structure. The structuring of the new building may not be able to utilize any of the structuring of the existing building (e.g., for support of floors). Thus, for some projects, this integrity factor may mean that the new structure is, from a design perspective, a separate structure that happens to abut an existing structure.

A NEW STRUCTURE

More freedom of design is generally possible when a completely separate structure is contemplated. However, constraints affecting structural matters are still evident.

If the project is a totally new structure, then any structure is possible, provided local codes and regulations are met. However, if the new structure is to be located near other buildings, any guidelines on the style of those facilities may have to be adhered to. Also, if the new structure is to be located adjacent to an existing medical building, style may be restricted.

Local traditions or preferences may also affect the type or style of structures that can be built in a particular area or region. Some research into this factor could be time and effort well spent.

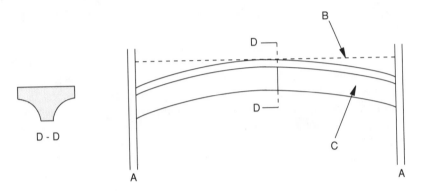

A = COLUMN OR WALL BEARING
B = LEVEL FLOOR
C = PRESTRESSED SLAB OR 'T' SECTION
        (EXAGGERATED FOR ILLUSTRATION PURPOSES)

Figure 6-1. Precast concrete.

TYPES OF STRUCTURES

The three basic structural materials used today are concrete, steel, and wood. Each has advantages and disadvantages. Each can be used alone or in conjunction with the other. Because of its combustibility, wood is quite restricted when used for structural purposes in health care facilities. A general discussion of some of the more popular structural configurations follows.

Concrete (Poured in Place)

In most cases, concrete poured in place will be reinforced concrete of either slab band, slab, or pan slab with concrete columns and beams (Figs. 6-1, 6-2). For one- or two-story structures, a wall-bearing condition with concrete slabs and beams might be considered. A structural engineer should be retained to assist in determining the best and most economical selection.

Concrete has proved to be the most versatile material for health care facilities since it gives good fireproofing without additional messy material, it allows holes to be located almost anywhere for utilities, and it facilitates any future alterations.

Steel

A steel skeleton is the next best selection for health care facilities since it can be erected relatively fast, and it allows work to proceed quickly for other trades. However, it does require fire-proofing with a fire-resistive material. This can be messy.

Steel structures can be combined with concrete floor slabs of both precast and poured types (discussed later). A metal deck of a ribbed nature with concrete topping can also be used. Holes for utilities will require special attention and additional reinforcement, since holes for this type of construction do not easily lend themselves to future relocation.

Steel beams and columns require a preorder time. Because delivery time can vary, this has to be taken into consideration.

Concrete (Precast)

There are several types of precast systems. The precast post and beam (columns and beams) with either precast slabs or poured concrete slabs can be used. Precast and prestressed floor and roof slabs can also be used.

> **NOTE:** Precast and prestressed types cannot be cut for utilities to pass through. Holes for utilities must be designed into this type of system.

Precast slabs have a camber (i.e., a curved rise due to the prestressed reinforcing) that must be taken into account (see Fig. 6-1).

This type of system lends itself best to parking garages, bridges, and buildings with few utility holes.

Wood

The wood structure is very easy to build. However, in most instances, fire safety restrictions limit the height of such a structure to a one-story, isolated building. Other fire-resistive considerations are necessary, such as treated wood, ceiling and partition construction, and exiting conditions.

Local building officials and fire prevention officers must be consulted before serious consideration is given to the use of wood.

Masonry Structure (Concrete Block or Brick)

A wall-bearing masonry structure might be considered for one-, two-, or three-story buildings. It can be combined with concrete slabs or precast slabs. Both exterior walls and interior partitions can be wall-bearing (i.e., the walls carry the load in place of

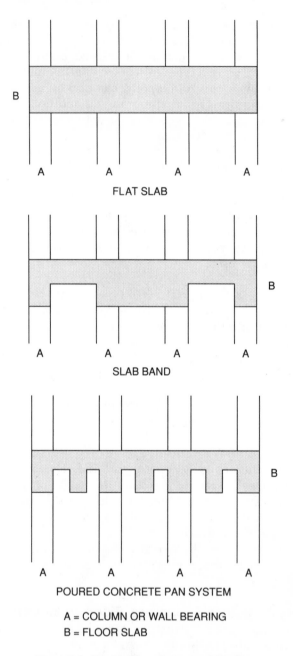

FLAT SLAB

SLAB BAND

POURED CONCRETE PAN SYSTEM

A = COLUMN OR WALL BEARING
B = FLOOR SLAB

Figure 6-2. Combination of structural framing.

beams or columns). This method is best for such buildings as nursing homes, dormitories, and some utility-type structures because of its cost and ease of construction.

Combinations

One or more of the preceding types of structures can be combined, though a structural engineer must be consulted in the process. As with the other types of structures discussed, the requirements for strength, fire-resistive level, and versatility of use (to do the job for the particular project) must be met. Figure 6-2 shows some of the more common combinations used.

THE SKELETON

The foregoing discussion should be studied carefully because the most often forgotten part of a building is the structure (skeleton), or frame as a whole. In the past, it has been covered up (or over) with brick, glass, gypsumboard, or other materials. Architects and designers went to great lengths to conceal it from view. In recent years, however, efforts have been made to leave some portions of the framing exposed for architectural purposes. Instead of being just functional, the skeleton has become aesthetic as well.

Whether or not the skeletal element of the facility is exposed, it is a part of the building that is very important from another aspect: it holds everything up! The right method of structure for a particular building is essential. It thus affects, and is affected by, several factors, among them:

1. Size of the building. It is the frame that determines the height, width, and depth of a building.

2. Subground conditions. What exists below the ground affects what can be built above the ground.

3. Use of the building. Average loads, heavy loads, and mixed loads affect the skeleton and size.

4. Location of the building (this relates to items 1 and 2). When the total square footage of the area needed or desired is determined for the project, how it will be arranged (structured) determines in part where it will or can be located.

5. Availability and cost of material. Although any material can be shipped anywhere, one type of material may be more economical than others for a particular locale. For a large project this could amount to millions of dollars.

6. Space available. The size of the plot of land may force (constrain) design to go more vertical than desired as well as impact on the type of structure possible.

7. Time required to build or the time within which the building is desired. Different frames take different amounts of time to erect — not just days, but months.

All of the preceding factors must be taken into consideration before a particular design is selected.

In this regard, one of the major items that is given too little attention during skeleton selection time is the amount of space consumed by the frame, columns, beams, and bearing walls. Their size and final interior location can be disconcerting to those who will be working in an area and who will have to take into account something they had not expected: for example, a 2-square-foot column or a 10-by-10-foot room instead of an 11-by-11-foot room.

Another related skeletal issue is the space requirements peculiar to health care facilities and their effect on framing. Aside from the usual constraints a large lecture hall presents, health care facilities can have three distinctive requirements. The first is an operating room (or generally several), which cannot have any columns running through it. Operating rooms for major surgery are becoming larger and larger because of the growing amount of equipment necessary to support the types of procedures now being done. Second, there is also the need in some areas to support very heavy equipment (e.g., CAT scanners, magnetic resonance imaging systems, lithotriptors). Provisions for these bulky devices must be taken into account at the skeletal stage. The third distinctive requirement is the constantly changing and advancing world that health care facilities find themselves in today. The ability to adapt, and not box in, an area has to be kept in mind so that future changes may be possible without major structural redesign. (This third item is difficult to define precisely; it is included here only as a marker for consideration.)

THE SKIN

The outer walls, or skin, that envelops the skeleton of a structure may vary with location, with the desire or the aesthetic nature of the owner, and with the skill of the architect. As with the interior structure, there are certain fire-resistive codes that must be enforced.[2] These are for material, glass (window) size, type of adjacent structure permitted, and fire zone levels (areas of the city or town as designated by local authorities).

NOTES

1. Refer to NFPA 101, Life Safety Code, and NFPA 220, Standard on Types of Building Construction, for details.

2. NFPA 101, NFPA 220, and state and local fire and building codes apply.

CHAPTER 7

Selecting the Four
Major Consultants

There are all types of specialists in the world, for all kinds of purposes, yet there are no all-purpose specialists or consultants.[1] Thus, no one consultant can possibly be so knowledgeable as to provide an administrator or governing board with all the assistance needed during the building of a health care facility (and some assistance is necessary, no matter how large the institution[2]).

Of the many types of specialists, only four major ones are discussed here:[3] the health care facility consultant, the financial consultant, the architectural consultant (sometimes referred to as the architect/engineer), and the construction consultant (sometimes referred to as the contractor).

Before the special roles, limitations, and criteria for selection of each consultant are discussed, their similar characteristics and functions are presented.

GENERAL CONSIDERATIONS
Commonalities
The definition of a consultant is one who gives professional advice or service. Each of the aforementioned individuals meets that definition since each is paid to provide specified services. It should be noted that because of this professional status, they are also very much accountable for their advice.

Generally, prospective consultants are interviewed to determine if they meet the specific needs of the project. This entails an "impression factor," or how well they impress owners initially when being interviewed. However, owners should not base their decisions exclusively on the interview. Although each prospective candidate can be expected to stress his or her expertise and past accomplishments on projects similar to the one being proposed, owners should not hesitate to request a list of all past projects. Contacting some or even all persons who worked with the candidate should provide a better picture of how well the candidate has been able to work in different situations. The ability to work with all kinds of persons is a vital qualifying mark of a good consultant.

Contracts, Fees, and Details

With respect to fees, a contract is generally negotiated in which the following are specified:

- A description and extent of work to be performed

- When reports, if any, will be due

- When work is to be completed

- The amount of money that will be paid for work and when and how remuneration for such work will be paid

Although all consultants are paid by a facility, they do not receive any of the normal benefits employees may be receiving (e.g., health insurance, paid vacation time, sick leave). This may seem obvious, but clarification of the following details may be necessary during negotiations, depending on the work involved:

1. Access to and use of owner's facilities, equipment, parking spaces, even staff

2. Access to and use of facilities during working and nonworking hours

3. Extent of accident coverage and other insurance

4. Extent and use of utilities (e.g., electricity, water, heat)

5. Location of any working trailers (architect/engineer, and contractor)

6. Location for storage of materials (contractor)

7. Arrangement for delivery of, and storage prior to use of, material

8. Disposal of trash

9. Ownership of salvagable material

Order of Selection of Consultants

Which consultant is hired first will depend on the internal resources of the facility, the amount of liquid assets available, and
the method of construction it intends to use. The first two factors
are finance related and must be totaled against the approximate
cost envisioned for the project. If the financial position is strong
then more emphasis can be placed on retaining the architect/en-
gineer and construction consultants than on the financial
consultant.

The third factor, method of construction, makes the order of
selection of consultants more complicated. Since the method of
construction itself determines the order, the most common
methods are listed subsequently, with a description of the general order of selection of consultants associated with each. (These
methods are discussed in Chapter 14.)

> **NOTE:** This selection of construction method occurs
> later, after any preconstruction planning by a health
> care facility consultant that might be used.

Traditional Bid Method. The financial consultant and architect/
engineer should be selected at approximately the same time: the
former to determine financial constraints and the latter to determine program (physical and operational) parameters. The contractor (builder) is selected by the bid process.

Construction Manager Method. The construction manager (in
most cases, also the builder), the architect or engineer, and the
financial consultants should be selected at approximately
the same time: the construction manager to advise and monitor
the physical building costs, the architect and engineer to determine program (physical and operational) parameters, and the
financial consultant to determine overall (facility and government) financial constraints. If the project is to go to bid, the
contractor is selected at this time as well.

"Fast-Track" Method. The contractor, financial consultant, and
architect or engineer are all hired at the same time. This method
involves all the same persons as the construction manager

method but allows construction to proceed without a bid system (e.g., subtrades are usually bid). It also allows construction to start prior to completion of all architectural and engineering documents. All consultants must thus be in constant communication in order for this method to have any chance of staying within original estimates.

"Not to Exceed Price" (or Guaranteed Maximum Price) Method. The contractor, financial consultant, and architect and engineer are all hired at the same time. However, the contractor will exert the most pressure because he or she, as the price setter, has to control the financial level of the project in greater detail.

In each of these methods, a clerk of the works is hired by the owner just before construction begins to monitor the building process for the owner.

Finally, various combinations of construction methods will cause a need for overlapping of the preceding methods. However, it is advised that all required consultants be retained in the earliest stages of any project to establish a strong working team.

A closer look will now be taken at these four key individuals or possibly companies. (Often a company or portion of a company is retained because of the extensiveness of project.) The specific services each provides will also be examined, as well as specific factors that owners should be aware of when selecting each consultant.

HEALTH CARE FACILITY CONSULTANT

A search for assistance in organizing the enormous amount of work required by most construction or renovation projects can start by retaining the services of a health care facility consultant. This person must be knowledgeable of the many details that have to be considered before even a commitment to build is made. The services of this person may not always be necessary, however, depending on the extent of the project and how much homework a facility is able to do on its own (i.e., through the expertise and/or experience of the facility staff).

There are many health care facility consultants in the field today, each with varied expertise. A careful selection should thus be made because of the importance of this individual in getting a project started efficiently. Some qualifications or abilities of health care facility consultants include:

1. A knowledge of the *political atmosphere* in the region with regard to health care facilities and their construction. Knowing whom to talk with is vital.

2. A grasp of the *Certificate of Need (CON)* situation in the region.

3. An ability to plan the *best approach* for a project in order to optimize receiving approval to carry out the project.

4. In connection with item 3, the ability to make *space plans* for a floor or building with respect to CON priorities. This would include determining the value of an expansion or renovation for any existing department(s), as well as the interrelationship and effect of changes on other departments.

Health care facility consultants, in a sense, act as initial guides, advising on a variety of fronts. If their strength happens to lie in a particular area, such as finance, they might continue as the financial or other applicable consultant as plans become firmer. Otherwise, these strategic planners are generally retained only during the initial phase of a project, though sometimes periodically thereafter for project review purposes.

> **NOTE:** The preceding discussion may imply that a facility need hire only this consultant to the exclusion of others. Also, some health care facility consultants might even claim that they can do it all. Both of these contentions are false. No one consultant can be so thoroughly knowledgeable of the entire construction process as to preclude the need for other consultants. The process of building or renovating a health care facility crosses or involves too many disciplines for one person to be an expert in each. The health care facility consultant must therefore be willing and able to work with other consultants, particularly the architect/engineer, and, if the construction manager method is used, with the contractor.

FINANCIAL CONSULTANT

As noted in Chapter 3, money is necessary to build or renovate anything, including a health care facility. Because of the amounts involved even in adding a small wing to an existing small facility, the management of money is very important to make sure a facility obtains the most money possible at the lowest cost and utilizes money in the most advantageous way while construction is in progress. This, then, is the rôle of a financial consultant: to optimize the acquisition and utilization of funds.

As part of this role of managing funds for a project, the financial consultant should be able to analyze the financial condition of the institution. This analysis is important so that the cash flow of the project (if the project is a new addition) does not disrupt established cash flow. In addition, it is important that the expected cash flow of the new facility integrate efficiently with any existing cash flow system. Knowing how an institution operates financially is thus a necessity.

In retaining the services of a financial consultant, a facility should conduct a solid investigation into his or her prior record, particularly with regard to health care projects of the type contemplated. How many years has the consultant been in this field? Does he or she have an updated knowledge of health care construction in the owner's state? Is he or she aware of the ever-changing cost levels for the type of project being considered (i.e., projects done several years ago have to be cost-updated, taking into consideration inflation, market conditions, construction time, and actual value). Knowledge of the Determination of Need and Certificate of Need processes and requirements is mandatory.

A financial consultant must also be thoroughly versed in tax laws—both federal and those for the state(s) in which construction is being done and headquarters are located (if different). A sizable amount of money might be unnecessarily paid in taxes if tax laws are not understood completely.

> **NOTE:** If a facility had no plans to build but suddenly came into enough capital to renovate, add a new service, or otherwise make modifications, much time and energy will be saved in actually starting a project since the fund-raising phase will not have to take place. As a result, the need for a financial consultant may be minimal or nil initially.

ARCHITECT/ENGINEER

It is not easy to select the man, woman, or group who will be responsible for creating the theme and atmosphere of a structure or renovated area. That person must translate ideas, traditions, preferences, and other abstractions into plans that, when implemented, will somehow physically reflect those ideas. Since the results cannot be fully judged until the project is essentially complete, the most crucial portion of the design phase becomes the translation step, for which an architect is responsible. Owners or administrators must therefore have a lot of confidence in the architect they select. This can make the selection of the architect very difficult.

It should also be noted that, when selecting an architect, one is also selecting a team. That is, the selection of an architect includes engineers who will be assisting the architect during the design stage. These engineers are necessary for their in-depth knowledge of heating, ventilating, air conditioning; electricity; structure; plumbing; and landscaping. In some cases, these engineers can be hired separately, but this can be a source of much aggravation since an architect needs the support of engineers in the design of a facility. If engineers are hired separately, different desires and methods of design might cause undue friction, resulting in a less than satisfactory working team.

Who Are Architects/Engineers?

One could say that architects are artisans, painting and sculpting in concrete, glass, steel, or wood on a scale that people can live in, work in, visit, or travel across. Unlike painters or sculptors, however, architects are under many more constraints and rules in following their vocation. These constraints come from the people (owners) desiring the structure their way; from regulations of various enforcing authorities that exercise control over all aspects of building and operating health care facilities; and from the fact that people will be more than looking at the results— they will using the building, or crossing the bridge (i.e., the results have to be functional for humans).

Architects must or should ask everyone involved with the project what they feel they want. Unfortunately, building a structure must be envisioned; one cannot experience the new structure unless exactly what is desired already exists somewhere. This is not very probable, however, human nature being what it is. So an architect must try to convey, in manners understandable to nonarchitects, what those ideas and desires for a structure translate into for design purposes. This can be in the form of scale models, sketches, renderings, detailed drawings, and/or computer imaging.

Constraints on Architects/Engineers

As mentioned, there are a variety of constraints and boundaries under which architects and engineers must operate in carrying out the wishes of owners. These include:

1. The geology and geography of the land, and thus the maximum load possible for the land

2. Local building ordinances, and thus the maximum dimensions of any new structure

3. Environmental influences (e.g., the location in the country; the type of weather that can be expected; environmental regulations)

4. Building and fire codes (to be discussed in Chapter 11)

5. Money (there is always a budget!)

One aspect of items 2 and 4 is how much influence regulations have over the design of a structure. Some critics say that codes and standards restrict design, whereas others say that they are able to design to code and still produce desired results. As will be discussed in Chapter 11, regulations are promulgated in the public interest. Thus, while they may impact on design, they also serve to make a building safer both during normal operating conditions and in emergencies. There is little incentive, then, to ignore these regulations in designing structures. Designing to codes and standards, in fact, helps reduce liability.

Regulations are also a reason why architects are not anxious to seek waivers from the requirements contained in codes. Waivers are statements that something else is considered equivalent to that which is contained in the regulation. Waivers also become the responsibility of the architect since he or she is the one who states that the "something else" is equivalent or nearly equivalent to the regulation itself.

Methods of Selection

There are several places to begin the selection process. One is attending architectural exhibitions. There, architects display models, plans, photographs, and other representations of their works. Names of architects can be obtained, as well as comparisons made of the works of each. Owners can even speak directly with architects to get a better understanding of an architect's philosophies, styles, and fees as well as personality.

Another way to start can be obtaining a list of architects from such organizations as the American Hospital Association and the American Institute of Architects (AIA). Usually, some description of architects and their styles is included. From these listings and descriptions, owners can begin to focus on those architects that appear promising.

A third way is to tour other health care facilities that have completed projects similar to the one contemplated in order to decide if the themes, layouts, traffic patterns, and other details are of the type desired. This method, however, should be tempered with the realization that the owner and architect may not have been able to agree on everything, that budgetary constraints may have altered what was really desired, and that the owner may not want to discuss difficulties that might have affected the final outcome. But standing in and touring facilities will help owners visualize and better explain to architects what they desire for their facility.

As to actually hiring an architect, several methods exist. One is a formal architectural competition. In this method, several architects are given the same information on the facility's needs and desires and are asked to prepare a design in the form of sketches, models, preliminary drawings, or some other form of presentation. Monetary remuneration is provided each architect for his or her efforts, and the amount may be significant. This method requires considerable effort to coordinate in order to make the competition fair. To that end, the AIA has prepared a resource guide, *Handbook of Architectural Design Competition*, on conducting an architectural competition (see Bibliography).

An architectural competition is a useful way to gain insight into the ideas and concepts of several architects. However, its applicability for heath care facilities may be limited because architectural competitions emphasize the overall design of a project, particularly exterior shapes and themes. For health care facilities, internal functioning is as important as the exterior design, but firm internal plans are very costly. In recent years, however, with competition affecting even health care facilities, concern for image has been increasing. As a result, owners have had to use every advantage possible to attract patients and staff.

The appearance of the facility is one part of that image and is thus gaining more attention during the design phase.

Another method is making a *short list* of potential architects, which is usually limited to three or four entries, and then inviting each one for a personal interview and presentation before a small group from the facility's administration or board. This will indicate how desirous each is of doing the project, the ability of each to do what the administrator, board, and owner want, and what each has to offer in order to do the best job. It will give board members and others the opportunity for direct dialogue with the architect and his or her associates. This opportunity to see if communication will be easy is very important on projects that generally involve much time, effort, and expenditures of money.

Whatever method is used, it is important that each architect be given a comprehensive outline and narrative about the proposed project: what is desired, who desires it, when it is desired, and so on. Conversely, information is needed from each prospective architect in order to make the best decision for the facility: for example, their previous work, particularly in the health care field; their philosophy on health care architecture; their general fees and schedule. Because the health care industry needs sophisticated building systems, it requires experienced designers.

In connection with experience, a relatively new question being asked of architects is the extent to which they use computers to assist them in the production of architectural drawings, cost estimating, and scheduling. High-power computers are now available that can process the large amounts of data related to construction projects. Designs can be analyzed more thoroughly for structural soundness and efficiency using such systems as computer-aided design software. Cost estimates can be more accurate utilizing computers. Asking questions about computer use will indicate how progressive and open an architect is to new ideas. (For further discussion on drawings, see Chapter 12.)

Fees

Finally, the subject of fees must be discussed early and thoroughly in the selection process so that no costly surprises occur later, when a misunderstanding on money could jeopardize the progress of the entire project. (See Chapter 3 for a discussion of finances.)

The AIA formerly advised on fee levels, and architects adhered to them. However, as the field became inundated with health care architects, fees began to vary widely. Unlike in other fields, competition did not generally reduce costs because the services desired of, and provided by, architects varied widely.

As a result, today, for new construction, fees for architects/ engineers vary from 6 to 10 percent of the cost of a project. As the size of the project increases, the fee in most instances will decrease (percentage-wise, not in actual dollars).

For renovation of existing structures, fees vary from 11 to 16 percent, depending on the complexity of the project. The percentage is slightly higher in this area than for new construction because much more investigation is required, and plans must be drawn up prior to doing work. As a result, in renovation work, gutting an area or building can actually be less costly in many cases than trying to revise existing partitions, run new wiring, install or modify ductwork, and so on.

For either project, new or renovation, costs for such items as travel, lodging, printing, and telephone calls will be billed separately. Although these costs can be only roughly estimated, by having them itemized, owners will be paying only for actual expenses incurred. Thus, architect's/engineer's fees, both the compensating and itemized charges, should be thoroughly discussed before an agreement or contract is signed.

It is important to select an architect who is right for the particular project. Appropriate experience, coupled with the prospects of a good working relationship with the administration and staff of the existing facility or with the owners planning a new facility, is essential.

CONSTRUCTION CONSULTANT

Selection of the construction consultant, or contractor, can be just as difficult as selection of the three previous consultants, even though money may have been secured and a design agreed on and approved. The wrong contractor can make the project take longer than anticipated or end up costing much more than expected.

There are several types of construction methodologies in use today. The type chosen for the project will in turn influence the selection of the contractor since different selection criteria exist for each type of construction.

Types of Construction and Their Impact on Selection of Contractor

The types of construction impacting on the selection of a contractor can be grouped into three major categories: bid method, construction manager method, and design/build method. (See Chapter 14 for a discussion of construction methods.)

Each method should be studied and compared to the others to determine which is best for the particular project. Factors that affect selection include the amount of liquid assets; the technical capability of owners, and how much they want to be involved in or control actual construction; and how fast owners want the project completed. Each method, then, involves varying amounts of preparation time.

A *straight bid* method will produce a bid from several contractors (or builders). The low bid will be chosen, given no other influencing factors. If this is a private project (i.e., no government funds involved), the list of bidders can be limited to or selected from a group of contractors in a selected area. Bidders should be financially sound, have experience in the health care field (optimally in projects similar to the one being contemplated), and be able to provide a schedule that fits into the facility's building program. If this is a public project (i.e., government funds are involved), a wider bid list is required by law, and owners have much less control in making the final selection.

If a *construction manager* method is used, selection of the construction firm will take place at the same time as the selection of the architectural/engineering firm. The construction manager will serve as a guide to determining the cost of construction. The construction manager may also become the prime contractor for construction of the project, although it is not required that the construction manager do so; the construction manager may act only as the cost consultant. The selection of this consultant will follow the same procedures as used for the selection of the architect/engineer, except that there will be a strong emphasis on prior records of cost control.

The consultant in the *design/build method* is a combination of architect/engineer and contractor. If this method is used, a more thorough investigation of the various firms' prior record is advised. The selection of this type of consultant may appear to be less costly than that of others initially, since the one consultant will be performing two tasks with which he or she is thoroughly familiar. However, the cost of both designing and building will be included eventually. Thus, extra care is needed in the selection of this consultant.

Fees

Fees in connection with a construction consultant can be grouped into two categories: fees related to construction and fees paid directly to the construction consultant. (See also Chapter 16 for a discussion on final payments.) Depending on payment arrangements, the construction fees may be paid through the consultant.

Construction Fees. There are several ways fees can be paid.

First is a flat, agreed-upon fee for all work to be performed. A second is a percentage fee based on the cost of the project. This may entail many cost items that have to be identified prior to signing a contract. (With respect to these items, the major question to answer is whether they are to be included in the fee.) Examples of items would be fixed or movable equipment.

A third method is an upset fee based on the cost of the project. This type of fee will not exceed an agreed-upon figure and is used mostly for construction management projects that have construction costs guaranteed by a construction firm. In this case, if the project does cost less than estimated, the share of savings the contractor will receive is determined ahead of time.

> **NOTE:** In most cases the architect/engineer fees will remain based on the guaranteed figure.

Construction Consultant Fees. Several fee schedules are currently used for paying construction consultants, depending on the type of construction methodology used.

For the management portion of the consultant's responsibilities, construction management fees will vary from 4 to 6 percent, depending on the size and complexity of the project.

In place of a formal fee there can be a profit reflected on the tally sheets. This will vary from 5 to 10 percent, with an additional 5 to 10 percent of the first figure for employer's overhead and insurance. (The exact accounting of this should be identified in writing prior to the signing of a contract.)

In design/build projects, the fee or profit for both architect and engineer and contractor may be included in the total quoted price of construction and not known to the owner.

CAUTION: Be sure to know all items included in every contract, and do not be reluctant to ask questions. If an unfamiliar term is used, ask about its exact meaning. It is better to ask today than pay more later.

NOTES

1. The term *consultant* is used as is generally understood in the business world: someone, not on staff, who is paid to do a specific task. In some areas of the country, other terms for this person may be used.

2. The only exception might be a large corporation whose business is the designing, building, and running of its own network of hospitals, nursing homes, other facilities. These companies would employ not only the four major consultants discussed but also other consultants, plus the administration, medical, nursing, and support personnel to operate the facility once it is built.

3. An owner might retain similar consultants during a project, either for a second opinion or because of the uniqueness of a particular aspect of the project.

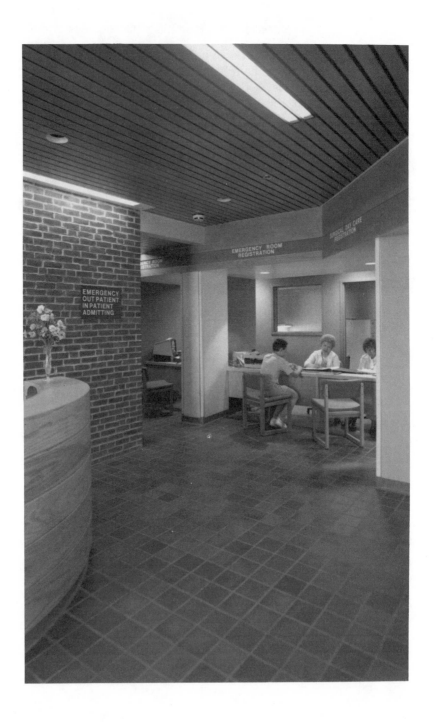

Part II

The Design Stage

CHAPTER 8

Evaluation of Existing and New Facilities and Operations

As discussions become more serious about the building of a new structure or the renovation of an existing facility, there will come a time when a hard look at any existing facilities and operations, as well as ideas for new facilities and operations, becomes necessary. There is no specific time this analysis should commence, but the more time spent analyzing what is happening and/or what is desired, the more likely the resultant project will fulfill the needs of the institution and community it is serving.

The level of detail of the evaluation matrix depends on the extent of the project. The evaluation can cover any or all of the following:

- Existing facilities—the current physical condition of any structures

- Existing operations—what activities are currently taking place

- Existing facilities for existing operations—when only renovations are contemplated

- Existing facilities for new operations—when renovations are for changes in operations as well

- New facilities for existing operations—when an expansion of current operations is contemplated

- New facilities for new operations—when creation or addition of new services in a new structure is contemplated

This may seem to complicate matters, but these are the possibilities that can exist. To be sure, not all these possibilities will be applicable for a particular project (e.g., a new facility in a new location will involve only the last possibility), but at least several of the preceding possibilities should be examined in some depth in order to learn and decide which one or more would be best for owners in terms of cost, convenience and/or inconvenience, and service to staff, patients, and the community.

First, it is necessary to look at several factors that need to be considered in any evaluation—the "who," "when," and "what" of an evaluation.

WHO SHOULD DO THE EVALUATION?

Because of the huge array of factors and influences involved, it is not possible for one person to know everything about evaluating an existing or projected health care facility. The combined expertise and views of many are necessary and should be solicited. The following is a description of the major persons who should be involved in any evaluation. Their involvement should be supplemented by that of even more specialized experts as a situation warrants.

- The *owner*. This is the person(s) legally responsible for the facility or project. Depending on the extent of the project, this could involve the administrator of the facility, or one or more of his or her assistants who have been given authority to act on behalf of the administrator; or the chairperson of the board of directors, or members of the board as designated by the chairperson. There should always be someone whose only function is watching out for the interests of the governing board of the facility.

- The *financial consultant*. This person must have experience with the Certificate of Need (CON) and/or Determination of Need (DON) approval process and with feasibility studies. He or she must also be given access to all the financial capabilities of the institution or owners in order to determine what kind of financial commitments are possible. Obviously, the financial consultant must have the complete trust and confidence of the owner. (See Chapter 7 for a more complete description of the financial consultant and his or her role in the building process.)

- The *architect/engineer*. This person should be experienced in analyzing data and preparing reports that detail the approaches that can be taken to meet the needs of the facility. He or she must be able to provide accurate pros and cons for each possible approach so that the owner, who is ultimately responsible for selecting the approach, has the most complete set of information to make that selection. The architect/engineer here does not necessarily have to be the same architect/engineer described in Chapter 7, who is retained to design the facility. This evaluation stage is just that—a time to evaluate various approaches—and the architect/engineer should be involved at this time.

These three persons or groups cannot and should not make the evaluation in a vacuum. It is critical that input from all staff (for an existing facility) be solicited and utilized. These are the persons who will have to work in the structure and environment created, so their thoughts should be considered carefully on such subjects as patient movement and routine patient care, steps to take in a medical or facility emergency, equipment and space requirements for medical services to be provided, present and future storage needs, and trends in medical care. For a new facility, comments from staff members in other similar facilities should be sought.

It takes many persons doing different tasks, in addition to treating patients directly, to make any health care facility operate efficiently and effectively. These activities range from regulating building temperature and humidity, maintaining surgical supplies, and preventing infections through washing and cleaning of the facility to ensuring the functioning of physiological monitors and sending out accurate statements of accounts.

WHEN SHOULD THE EVALUATION BE DONE?

There are actually two evaluation periods that need to be considered—an informal one and a formal one.

An informal evaluation period can be considered the planning phase of a long-range plan (LRP). This is a 5- to 10-year plan of what, among other things, owners believe should be built, either onto existing structure(s) or completely separate. By going through this exercise, owners can estimate what services, and thus what facilities, a community needs and approximately when the community needs them.[1]

When activities or conditions, as projected in the LRP, begin to take place, a formal, in-depth evaluation, as described in the next section, can be initiated. A detailed evaluation of what is currently taking place and what is possible to undertake will be conducted. Given the lead time required for most projects, the three major evaluators noted above need to be quickly rallied and allowed to begin their detailed assignments. Otherwise, the cost in terms of time will quickly evaporate the ability to meet the needs of the community.

WHAT SHOULD BE EVALUATED?

To properly evaluate an existing facility, a complete architectural, mechanical, and electrical survey is needed. To do this, the following questions should be answered as part of this evaluation:

- Is there a physical need for such spaces as more operating rooms, patient bedrooms, treatment rooms, storage areas, or service areas?

- Is there a functional need to rearrange space for more efficient utilization of space and/or to lower operating cost per patient?

- Is there an update need to replace antiquated equipment or to install patient or environmental control equipment of new technology (either of which may require more space) or to reflect new fire, safety, environmental requirements or technology (e.g., installation of a new sprinkler system, replacement of old windows)?

Another fundamental issue is whether the existing facility is worth retaining or renovating, sentiments not withstanding. For some projects, it may not be necessary to pursue this issue—for example, if there are not sufficient funds to replace the existing structure; but for other situations, it may be necessary—for example, if the cost to upgrade or rearrange appears to exceed the cost of adding new space.

Thus, an existing facility must be surveyed from a practical approach to determine the status of space, structural condition, code compliance, plant utility, and medical requirements. Each department must be surveyed to determine what its projected needs are; this must be correlated with the whole facility. Is the department functioning up to its capabilities? Is equipment being overtaxed or undertaxed?

Evaluations for a new facility are very different but in some ways easier, since the issue of existing activities (or what to do about them) is not a factor. The adequacy of the site in terms of the needed size can be decided. The ease of access can be studied. All the requirements or influences noted in other chapters can be followed (i.e., the various fire, safety, building, and health codes; the newest structural technologies). A more accurate cost estimate is possible since the problems of an existing facility or of maintaining current activities do not have to be considered.

WHAT IS TO BE BUILT?

After evaluating current facilities and operations and the possibilities for new facilities and operations, how does one decide what is to be built? A simple answer can be whatever is needed most and is affordable. But the answer is more complicated than that. Some further considerations must be reviewed after the evaluation.

Community Needs

Until recently, the public advocate for determining community needs was the CON board, which decided if the project was needed. (Of late, the role of these boards has been declining because of a reduction in federal spending. See Chapter 2 for a discussion of this change.) Thus, where these boards are still effective, owners need to make some informal inquiries, as to whether CON approval is probable or doubtful in order not to waste money.

Economics

What is affordable—both to build and to operate? A complete picture of a facility's or owner's financial condition is critical. Financial capabilities can then be matched against the costs of several options that are usually generated from the evaluation.

Facility Needs (Structural and Operational)

This is a matter of setting priorities, developing various options against those priorities (via the evaluation), and then deciding which option can be implemented to meet the most needs. Two inputs that are very useful in this regard are consideration of the data from the three evaluators and an LRP outlining where owners want to be and what they want to be doing at various points in time.

A CHECKLIST: HOW TO SURVEY AN EXISTING FACILITY

To help readers see what should be evaluated, checklists have been included in the back of this book (Appendices A, B, C, and E). They are included to indicate all the items that must be reviewed. None of the questions should be skipped since each one is applicable to all facilities. If a question cannot be answered, it should raise the question of why it cannot be answered. A satisfactory answer should be indicated.

NOTES

1. Some states require a 5- to 10-year plan to be filed with the state.

CHAPTER 9

Architecture for New Facilities

After the evaluation of existing facilities and operations, the next step (although it can be initiated during that evaluation) is the design for the new wing or structure.[1] Preliminary ideas can be put to paper very early in the project, but serious designs should not be finalized until everyone has approved designs for the new structure or wing.

GENERAL CONSIDERATIONS

Design can be divided into two major categories: exterior and interior. Each has its own set of possibilities and constraints, which are basically the sum of what has been presented thus far—geography, zoning regulations, existing facilities, CON approval, money, needs, and priorities.

In addition, other structural factors, which affect all commercial structures, have to be taken into account. Some of these are applicable to any habitable structure, though health care facilities may require narrower limits or stricter controls. Other factors are purely the result of the structure's being a health care facility.

Factors affecting the design of any habitable structure include the number of elevators and stairways necessary; energy conversion techniques or requirements; owners' or administrators' preferences on a design; the amount and shape of land available; and zoning height regulations. Design considerations applicable strictly to health care facilities include corridor width enabling patient beds to be turned around; special air circulation requirements; a defend-in-place concept as opposed to immediate exiting in an emergency; and emergency electrical power not only for exiting in an emergency but also for continuing certain essential activities during an emergency.

All these factors form a kind of backdrop to what an architect can design in meeting the requests and needs of the individuals desiring a particular design for their building or renovation project.

THE EXTERIOR

The design of the exterior shape and appearance of a structure places an architect in his or her element and tests his or her creative abilities against the realities of funding limits, nonarchitectural preferences, and the requirements of authorities (government and nongovernment) having jurisdiction over health care facility design and operation. The exterior of a building is a functioning element of a building; it is concerned with what takes place within the building, in addition to keeping out, or allowing in, the weather (e.g., fresh air, sunlight). It is an envelope that everyone approaching the structure will see, and it will not fail to create an impression when entering.

As creators of structural impressions, architects are thus very concerned about that envelope: what it tries to say or convey and how well it succeeds in conveying or exhibiting that theme or impression. Unless the new structure is an addition to an existing building, about the only physical limitations on design are the laws of physics. For example, a cantilever can be only so long and still be a safe support. Possibilities for the exterior design of a building would thus be almost unlimited were it not for nonarchitectural constraints that must be taken into account: for instance, what materials are reasonably available; whether existing surroundings are a factor; and whether there are height restrictions.

In terms of size, which can have a bearing on exterior design, there is the practical matter of what functions are to be included in the new structure, how much space each will require, and how these functions are to be arranged. This last factor will be discussed further in the next section.

The existing surroundings can have a large impact on the exterior. They can be classified as either natural or manufactured. Is the land barren or wooded? Rocky or hilly? Or is the land between two skyscrapers? Further, will the architect have the opportunity to try to match the building to the land?

Planning the exterior of a new structure is thus an exercise in unlimited possibilities tempered by reality and economics.

THE INTERIOR

An entirely different set of possibilities and constraints prevail for the interior design of a health care facility. Here, the forcing functions on design can be grouped into two major categories: internal operational requirements and external regulations. The test in terms of design is how well these internal and external factors can be accommodated, while still producing an efficiently organized and operating building.

Interior design itself falls into two categories: function and aesthetics, both of which are important and must work together.

The traffic flow within the building is of prime importance. All functions are related. The public (i.e., visitors) must not interfere with in-house functions. Thus, main lobbies, waiting areas, gift shops, and coffee shops for the public should be located with great care so that no internal cross traffic is involved. The public, however, must have quick and direct access to the areas they seek — mainly inpatient bed areas — without crossing the other facility paths of travel. This can be accomplished by *dedicated* corridors or elevators that provide a path to an area, reducing the chance of getting lost or arriving at the wrong destination. Here is where another impression is made, the first having been the impression made when approaching the building. A designer's ability to create a feeling of a modern, clean, and trustworthy facility meets its first test in the public lobby. Color, furniture, plantings, skylights, wall materials, and lighting are equally important. This space should not be cramped to save a few dollars in so-called square footage costs.

The more often overlooked areas where aesthetics and function must be combined with thoughtfulness and care are the emergency and outpatient spaces. More often than not, these areas tend to be cold and sterile, with waiting areas crowded, often along corridor walls. Donated secondhand furniture somehow has a way of finding its way into these areas.

Great thought should be given to these first "patient approach" spaces. Most patients coming to these areas are accompanied by relatives or friends and are fearful of what may happen next; thus a clearly defined path of travel should be indicated so that the patient knows where to go upon entering, and such things as the location of the restrooms are readily evident. Even decor can be utilized to provide instructions.

Outpatient and emergency areas should be adjunctive, as should associated radiology and laboratory services. This does not mean, however, that the entire radiology and laboratory departments need be located in this area. These three areas are interconnected by function, since both patients and staff may flow from one to the other as a matter of daily use. Care should be taken, however, to prevent cross traffic yet, at the same time, make each area accessible. Again, simple, understandable signage, with print of readable size, should be incorporated in the decor. Often, signage is placed after the interior is already designed and end up creating more turmoil than needed.

The color and material of furniture and decoration, as well as the arrangement of lighting, are important to creating a feeling of trust and calm in the patient. Pleasant colors also provide a good environment for facility employees, as people work better in their presence.

Many other spaces in a facility need equal attention. Corridors can be color-coded. Inpatient bedrooms do not have to be stark to be clean. Furniture can fit a room both physically and aesthetically. There are good washable paints and other materials that can be used in a health care facility.

For working areas, it has been proved that certain colors foster better performance than others. Thus, laboratories, kitchens, administration spaces, and anywhere people sit or are detained for long periods require great thought to achieve a pleasant, and thus productive, work environment.

From room to room and one department to the other, good interior space planning is important to avoid cross traffic and long, roundabout corridors. Interior designers are specialists, whose major responsibilities are meshing color with function. They can be hired for any size of project since color and function concerns exist at every level—from a single room to an entire structure. (For more detail on space and functional relationships, see the subsequent section, Some Specifics: From the Outside to the Inside.)

Internal Operational Requirements

To fully account for internal operational requirements, an architect needs to know exactly what owners or operators desire, or have had approved, for their new wing or structure. The following are some examples of what needs to be reviewed and studied:

- Number of beds (if an inpatient facility)

- Number of private rooms

- Number of operating rooms and their type

- Number of treatment rooms

- Number of physician offices

- Description of operational practices (current as well as those desired)

- Description of services to be provided (medical, laboratory, plant, dietary)

- Administrative functions to take place in the new area

- The anticipated materials and goods for the new area (e.g., use rates; in-house storage requirements)

Useful checklists have been published by various groups, including the American Hospital Association, The Ritchie Organization, and the Department of Health and Human Services. They list building interior functions and the features necessary to support such function (see the Bibliography).

Some constraints must also be taken into account during this phase. Some are staff oriented, such as preference of location within the new building. Others are mandatory, such as patient sleeping rooms having outside windows, infectious areas being segregated, and hazardous laboratories being located as remotely as possible from patient areas.

There is also the projected flow pattern of people and goods in movement to be considered. This has an effect on the location of patients and staff.

All these items have to be translated by the architect: from items on a list to a drawing showing where items will be located; from individual drawings of areas to complete layouts of each floor; from drawings of each floor to complete drawings of the entire building. In a sense, a kind of living system is created: each part related to, and making possible, the whole. It is thus crucial that everything expected or desired to take place in the new structure be known and defined.

As these internal operational factors become firm, a space versus function (program) can be analyzed. Initially, this is done on a room by room basis, but eventually this analysis has to consider entire floors and even the whole building (depending on the extent of the project). All this effort is aimed at producing an internal design that maximizes space and function in order to meet the prime purpose of a health care facility: medical service to patients.[2]

Regulations

Some government and nongovernment regulations affect interior design in the same way that external influences affect exterior design.[3] For facilities receiving Medicare and Medicaid funds as payments, the U.S. Department of Health and Human Services has published *Guidelines for Construction and Equipment of Hospitals and Medical Facilities*. It contains recommended criteria that can affect interior design, such as handicapped accessibility within the building, criteria for nurses' stations, sizes of patient and treatment rooms, and the number of janitor closets per floor.

It is thus essential that all regulations that can influence the interior design of a facility be known by, or conveyed to, the architect.

Some Specifics: From the Outside to the Inside

We do not presume to tell any architect or administrator how his or her facility should be planned or designed. However, over the years, some ideas have developed about how facilities function best, given the needs of the facility. They are now elementary, but often overlooked, details.

A facility, for example, should have a well-defined entrance and exit roadway. There should be a separate service and delivery roadway and an easy turnaround for large trucks, fuel tankers, and laundry and food delivery trucks. If the facility is in a snow region, there should be additional space for snow to be piled.

Adequate parking is necessary to accommodate employees, doctors, nurses, visitors, patients, salespersons, and emergency vehicles. What is provided is often far too small. Many times, physical expansion of a facility is accomplished at the expense of the existing parking. Sometimes a parking garage must be built so that people do not have to park several blocks from the main entrance. Certainly, it does not help the handicapped or safety in general to force people to park great distances from the facility.

This peripheral area at first glance might seem unrelated to internal functions. However, if just getting to the lobby or outpatient entrance is a hassle, a poor impression has already been created.

Inside a facility, there are several lobby functions that must be clearly available to the patient or visitor. The main lobby should contain information and directional facilities, waiting space, gift and coffee shops, telephone spaces, and public restrooms. For operational efficiency, this lobby may also include cleaning and storage space and some administration offices. In large facilities, a fire control unit space may be best located there.

Any emergency and outpatient lobbies should have complete access (no barriers) for fast entrance for handicapped, stretchers, and others who may have difficulty maneuvering. In addition, control and information, a police data room, waiting spaces, public toilets, privacy spaces for patient data, and administration spaces should be considered for these two lobbies. Since patients in the main lobby often have to go to one of these two lobbies, all three lobbies should be interconnected to a degree. In small facilities, these lobbies can even be shared.

For emergency facilities, adequate ambulance spaces and technician areas must be provided.

The laboratory and radiology areas needed to service the emergency and outpatient departments should be adjacent, with an easy path to each established and identified. If the facility has a blood bank that accepts public donations, it should also be adjacent to the outpatient space.

Both outpatient and emergency areas should have a direct path to such places as admitting for surgery, special care, coronary care. The delivery room access for emergency maternity patients should also be a direct path from the emergency area. In essence, patients must go by the shortest and most direct path without going through or into departments.

The *major* radiology and laboratory departments might be an expansion of those in adjunct to emergency and outpatient departments, but this is not a necessity. Only those services for immediate emergency use need be directly adjacent to the emergency and outpatient departments.

Delivery of portable equipment (e.g., monitors, respirators, gas cylinders) to inpatient bedroom floors must be considered. In most cases, a clear, direct use of corridor and elevators must be considered.

Such adjunct departments as physical therapy and hydrotherapy, if used in conjunction with outpatient spaces, should also have direct access from the outpatient area to the department.

Elevators should be dedicated, if possible, to specific uses: public visitors, surgery patients, food and services. Elevator size is directed by code, either an American National Standards Institute standard or a state's department of public health or federal minimum construction standard. A check of governing authority must be made.

For sterile and clean rooms (e.g., delivery rooms, surgical suites), sterile and semisterile functions can be somewhat isolated. However, direct paths (without cross traffic) from the patient bed and return are absolute requirements. Sterile supplies must have a direct path to surgical areas, yet care must be taken that soiled material has no cross traffic with clean supplies. This also applies to the delivery of goods from the outside and for goods being distributed to other parts of the facility. This requisite can be a frustrating design problem and, if not carefully studied, a space consumer.

Day Surgery. An ever-growing department in hospitals is day surgery, where patients are operated on and released in the same day. This area should be adjacent to the outpatient area, so that some of the aforementioned areas, such as lobby, waiting room, recovery, and records, can be shared. The increased load, of course, should be taken into account. If the main surgical area is to be enhanced to accommodate day surgical procedures, however, then a direct connection is required to these other areas.

Food. The location of the dietary department of a facility needs considerable study. It must have good delivery access from the outside, combined with proper and adequate storage space. It must be able to service patients, employees, and visitors. It is not always easy to solve the problem of steering traffic to several locations, such as patient rooms, employee dining, and visitors' coffee shop. Dedicated elevators for food carts should be considered.

Services. Spaces for shops such as electric, plumbing, air conditioning, heat, woodworking, and laundry may be isolated, but again, access and delivery are important. In these areas, ceiling height is an important consideration. Most will require a minimum of 10 feet, with storage provided on interior mezzanine levels.

Environmental control spaces (e.g., boiler plants), electrical emergency spaces, air conditioners, air handlers, electric power distribution panels, and pumps may also be isolated. However, access of utility to these various spaces has to be considered.

The location of utility services spaces is not entirely of a linear nature. In high-rise facilities, an intermediate floor can be considered. An upper floor would also apply where ground floor space is at a premium. Locating air conditioners and air handlers on the roof is a common practice. However, some thought should be given to expanding the use of upper levels to include other services (e.g., storage, electrical distribution panels).

Disposal. Incinerator spaces may be isolated spaces with proper access for disposal of ash or unburnable trash.

> **NOTE:** A facility might consider using heat generation from trash incineration.

Patient Versus Nonpatient Areas. It is worth some thought to divide patient care and services into two noncrossing sections, so that all service spaces are on one side and patient-oriented spaces are on the other. This type of space and function planning is in use at the Frisbie Memorial Hospital in Rochester, New Hampshire, where public and patient access and ingress are from one end and services from the other end.

A facility that is dedicated to a specific medical and surgical specialty has design problems similar to those listed previously, but the traffic flow is simpler, as patient treatment is linear.

Clinics and nursing homes each have individual problems. However, the relation of one space to another is similar to that in hospitals and just as pertinent.

Requisite Items. The one common oversight in space planning is forgetting, in the initial program, the requisite items. These include:

- Janitor closets
- Duct space allowance (both vertical and horizontal)
- Plumbing run-outs (require depths and add ceiling problems)
- Stairway space
- Interconnection passages and corridors
- Storage space (there never is enough)
- Employee lockers, rest rooms, toilets

- Door swing interference
- Electric closets (particularly those beyond the main distribution panel)
- Telephone equipment rooms
- Data processing rooms
- Drinking fountains
- Special equipment storage for intensive care and cardiac care units and other specialized areas
- Wheelchair and litter storage spaces (emergency and outpatient areas)
- Handicapped toilets
- Volunteers' spaces, lockers, toilets
- Special services (e.g., flower rooms)
- Mail room
- Public relations offices
- Waiting space adjacent to administration offices
- Engineer's office
- Salespersons' waiting areas
- Patient record rooms (both on the floors and central)

CONCLUDING THOUGHTS

If design involves more than one area or department, or is for a specific type of facility, a room by room or space by space interview with *all* pertinent and affected personnel in the facility must be conducted. Many times, one hand does not know what the other has to contend with. It is not uncommon for each department to consider itself as the only one that needs more space.

The preceding review is not intended as a complete room by room space planner, but it is intended to alert readers to some commonly overlooked considerations.

In summary, interior space design and interior aesthetic design are so intertwined that one cannot be successfully done without the other.

NOTES

1. Design of architecture for existing facilities (i.e., renovations) is discussed in Chapter 10.

2. A general space by space (room by room) listing is provided in Appendix C for helping the reader understand what is involved during this period.

3. Regulations relative to fire and safety are discussed in Chapter 11.

CHAPTER 10

Architecture for Existing Facilities

In this book, architecture for existing facilities refers to any major renovation project that does not add floor space to an existing structure, but does require Certificate of Need (CON) board approval, or substantially alters the way the facility functions. In contrast to the considerable flexibility in design described in the previous chapter for existing facilities, the possibilities for originality in shape are restricted and constraints in remodeling space and organizing functions are more evident. Ingenuity, however, will play a significant role in how well the project succeeds or improves operations. The problem of limitation can thus be turned into an opportunity that challenges the resourcefulness of both owner and architect.

GENERAL CONSIDERATIONS

As for architecture for new facilities described in Chapter 9, renovation of existing facilities can be divided into two major design categories: exterior and interior. Each also has its own set of possibilities and constraints. However, exterior creativity is drastically reduced, unless the entire outer walls are to be replaced. Interior design is dependent, of course, on how much renovation is being proposed. For example, a complete gutting of an interior will create new building possibilities.

The work of the architect, however, is still considerably similar for existing facilities as for new facilities. He or she must meet the requests and/or needs of the individuals responsible for renovating the facility and have the design meet all the applicable codes, standards, and regulations.

THE EXTERIOR

Because no new floor space will be added to an existing facility, exterior design changes will therefore not involve creating a shape. Exterior work, however, can modify the *appearance* of the structure. Depending on the amount of money available, this can result in a new look with the installation of a new *skin* on the building.

Aside from cosmetic reasons, there are several major reasons for changing the appearance of the facility. The first is a need to repair those portions that are crumbling, weather-beaten, leaking, or otherwise deteriorating. If restoration to original design is not technically desirable or economically feasible, creating a new exterior (i.e., modifying the existing exterior appearance) may be a reasonable course of action.

The second, and more important reason, for exterior work is energy conservation: reducing oil, gas, and electricity usage. This work can be in the form of new thermal windows, a new skin that incorporates insulation, or addition of passive or active solar heating systems. A cost-payback study is necessary when these types of changes are being considered.

A third reason for exterior change is to allow access (and thus egress) for the physically handicapped. This, in fact, may be required by local regulations. Access for the handicapped would have to start from the property line and extend into the building. Thus, all approaches to the building, and at least one exterior door (depending on the size of the structure), would have to permit access by the physically handicapped.

> **NOTE:** Because probably all health care facilities by now have some handicapped access features, this issue is most applicable when a non–health care facility is converted into a health care facility.

In connection with exterior work, the grounds surrounding the structure should be reviewed for the following:

1. *Drainage*—changing the contour of the land to enhance water runoff away from the structure

2. *Landscaping*—to enhance the general appearance of the facility

3. *Parking and general access*—to provide the most convenient approaches to the facility

4. *Utility carriers* (e.g., electric poles)—These should be placed underground as much as possible to enhance appearance and reduce problems

5. *Service and delivery* approaches, roads, platforms

THE INTERIOR

Designing a new interior (either partial or total) for an existing facility has similarities to designing the interior for a new facility. Thus, the section on the interior in Chapter 9 should be reviewed. The difference in possibilities between new and existing facilities is the impact of the renovation project on the existing facility. The larger or more encompassing the project, the closer it will resemble a new facility project.

Internal Operational Requirements

If the project is the complete renovation and/or conversion of a building into a health care facility, then the same considerations listed in Chapter 9 are applicable. If the project is smaller then the possibilities for design are reduced and constraints are increased—that is, fewer options in design are possible. However, the complexities of internal operational requirements are concurrently reduced as the size of a project is reduced (i.e., the number of unknown variables is reduced).

External Regulations

Generally, the same external regulations affecting the design of new facilities are also applicable to existing facilities. There may be some allowances for existing buildings, however, since it may not be possible to do everything that is required of a new building. The extent to which an existing facility is brought up to new facility requirements depends on the amount and type of renovation work accomplished. If physical changes are minimal—that is, more cosmetic than structural—application of requirements for new facilities is less in many instances. Some codes differentiate between new and existing facilities (e.g., NFPA 101, Life Safety Code). If this is not the case, then waivers may have to be sought when the existing structure makes it impossible to meet requirements for new facilities.

Close attention to external regulations is important when renovating an existing facility. Personal judgment is often used, and necessary, in determining what regulations should be invoked.

CHAPTER 11

Meeting the Codes

The very word codes[1] is enough to trigger a knee-jerk negative reaction, hostility, or plain fear in some people. Many persons view codes as blockades to design, construction, or operation. On the other hand, others, having studied how the code-generating process functions and understanding the reasons behind requirements, use the codes and design according to them with few problems. Codes are part of our world. They consider it nearsighted to try to ignore or circumvent them. Why the gap?

In trying to answer this question and also exploring how codes impact on the building of health care facilities, we think brief historical overview might be helpful, if anything, to dispel some myths that exist even today.

Codes are a set of parameters, such as specifications, performance criteria, or installation requirements, that have been developed and judged as acceptable boundaries and minimum levels for safety and/or efficacy. They are restrictive because not everything that can be made or built will fit within those bounds, levels, or methods. They are also not absolute, as opposed to laws of physics, chemistry, or other disciplines. Rather, codes reflect what society is willing or able to accept or bear. They are subject to change as society's attitudes, economy, and values evolve. They are also subject to, or at least influenced by, technological changes or innovations.

Codes are not perfect. They can be and are changed as more information is learned about a procedure and how to codify it or mitigate any hazards associated with it.

Codes try to be unifiers without trying to inhibit progress. They are an attempt at describing what is acceptable at any given moment in history.

It should thus be remembered as the history of codes is discussed that the building industry, which has grown rapidly and become more complex in the last 40 years, would not have achieved its current level of quality or safety were it not for the use or enforcement of codes. Although the cost incurred as a result of following the codes cannot be ignored, neither can the cost of a building failure. The risk is too great in terms of human lives that will be occupying these buildings. Codes are part of a responsibility to the public to erect safe structures.

CODED HISTORY

Who or what develops codes? The answer lies in who perceives a need for their creation. There are hundreds of formal groups and organizations whose main purpose is producing codes for safety or efficacy. These include the National Fire Protection Association; the American Society for Testing and Materials; the American Society of Heating, Refrigeration and Air Conditioning Engineers; the American National Standards Institute; the model building groups; the U.S. government; and state agencies.

The real test for *voluntary* codes is the extent to which they are used: either voluntarily or through adoption and enforcement by some authority. Just like any other producer, the developers of these codes, of course, hope that their "product" will be used. Sometimes this use occurs voluntarily; that is, the code is followed, but no independent source checks to see if the user of the code is doing what the code calls for. Other times, an agency, organization, or company directs another company or facility to meet the requirements of a code, either for public safety or as a prerequisite for purchasing a product—for example, an insurance company that is insuring a facility; a state agency that is approving the construction of a building for occupancy; a store that is purchasing a product for resale. If a code developed by a nongovernment organization is adopted or referenced by a government agency, it assumes the posture of a regulation, though only by the agency's enforcing it and only within the jurisdiction of that group (e.g., for a state agency, only activities within the state; for a federal agency, anywhere in the country it has authority).

Many rules exist for producing codes, both those developed by regulatory agencies and those developed by nongovernment groups. In addition, in recent years, as the United States has become a more litigious society, developers of codes have added even more rules as their procedures have come under closer legal scrutiny. Despite a few glaring misdeeds, which have created much media coverage and congressional hearings and resulted in landmark lawsuits, by and large the people and organizations involved in developing the tens of thousands of nonregulatory (voluntary) codes have done a remarkable job[2]—and at no direct taxpayer expense.

Although it is an apparent incentive for manufacturers to participate in code development associated with their products, it is also to every sector's advantage to participate in the process. Private code developers recognize this natural self-interest of groups, and rather than try to ignore or resist it, they have taken the opposite tack and encouraged all affected interest groups to be represented. Although these code development systems are not perfect, they do have many checks and balances that prevent one interest group from dominating others.

WHO DEVELOPS CODES?

Generally, organizations develop the nonregulatory codes used to build health care facilities today. These can be multidisciplinary organizations with open or selected memberships (e.g., National Fire Protection Association, International Conference of Building Officials, Scientific Apparatus Makers Association) or organizations whose sole mission is the development of codes (e.g., American Society for Testing and Materials, American National Standards Institute). State and federal agencies either develop codes internally by the notice of public rule making (e.g., through notices in the Federal Register) or adopt codes by reference to codes developed by nongovernment organizations. The public rule-making process is still used, too.

Health codes are developed at the federal level through the Department of Health and Human Services and at the state level through public health departments. The codes for traffic control, utility usage, water, drainage, rights of way, zoning, handicapped access, and parking are usually developed by local authorities. (For a complete breakdown of codes, refer to Appendix A.)

WHO ENFORCES CODES?

Various government agencies and numerous nongovernment groups enforce all kinds of codes with regard to the building of health care facilities. The following is a list of groups in generally chronological order of participation, depending on the state in which the project is being done and on the extent of the project.

Certificate of Need (CON) reviewers in each state or locality (via the department of public health) approve plans using all codes as reference. They also inspect final construction using the same codes.

State public safety, and/or labor and industry, and its subdivisions review plans and final construction against codes it has adopted. In some states (e.g., Florida), a third party (architect/engineer) approved by the designated agency is required to review drawings—again, against codes adopted by the state.

Fire departments (e.g., the state fire marshal, local fire service, or both) review plans and inspect during construction against fire codes.

Building departments determine compliance against adopted codes. This department might also coordinate the enforcement of other local codes, such as zoning, utilities, traffic, and environmental.

Federal agencies enforce environmental codes, such as for wetlands, parks, forests, highways, and pollution.

The Joint Commission on Accreditation of Healthcare Organizations (JCAHO; formally JCAH) is a nongovernment organization that has developed and enforces medical, surgical, laboratory, and operational safety standards for hospitals and related facilities. JCAHO also references for enforcement purposes codes developed by other organizations, such as the National Fire Protection Association. (As noted elsewhere, the Health Care Financing Administration awards deemed status to facilities having JCAHO accreditation, thereby allowing Medicare and Medicaid payments to the facility.)

Insurance companies enforce codes, those developed by both others and the carrier itself. It is thus advisable to learn of any insurance requirements prior to design or construction.

Other federal agencies, such as the Veterans' Administration and the Department of Defense, enforce codes. Generally, they follow the codes used in the jurisdiction in which a facility is to be built, but since this is not always so, codes of these agencies should be investigated early in the design process.

WHO USES CODES?

Everyone involved in the design, financing, construction, or operation of a health care facility uses codes. There are no exceptions. It should be evident from the very concept of a project that the knowledge and use of codes are important factors in producing a structure that will protect the lives of the people within and around it. As has been implied several times, the earlier the codes are reviewed and their requirements and recommendations followed, the fewer the problems and the lower the costs later.

The extent of use of codes will vary, depending on the extensiveness of the project. In addition, use itself will vary since codes generally set minimum levels, and code developers cannot anticipate every possible construction problem or hazard for which a standard can be developed. Thus, those who use the codes should be aware of their limitations.

THE IMPACT OF CODES ON THE COST OF HEALTH CARE FACILITIES

How have codes affected the cost of a health care facility, and what have been the benefits from the added costs?

It is a fact that the level of loss of life from fires, disasters, and other accidents in health care facilities is now dramatically lower than it was 10 and 20 years ago. As a result, many point to this fact and say, "We have had no loss of life in our facility from fire, smoke, or faulty construction, so do we still have to comply with this or that requirement?" What is forgotten is that code requirements are the very reason for such low numbers of fatalities and incidents. This is very noticeable when comparing the records of pre-World War II buildings with those of post-World War II buildings, when code requirements were heavily changed to reflect increased fire and building science technology and the enforcement of these requirements was increased.

The arguments, which intimate that codes are the reason health care facilities cost so much, do not stand up under close examination.

First, the average current cost (depending on decor, finishing materials, services) to build a hotel is about $100 to $130 per square foot; an office building, about $60 to $80 per square foot; and an apartment building, about $95 to $125 per square foot. For an average 300-bed community hospital, the cost is about $100 to $160 per square foot. Thus, basic construction costs for a health care facility are not dramatically different from those for other types of occupancies. Technically, it is not legitimate to compare non-health care facilities with health care facilities since the "occupants" of health care facilities are not at all like the occupants of the other structures listed. The necessity for health care facilities to defend in place is more costly in terms of construction than an "exit immediately" philosophy for non–health care facilities.

Second, there are trade-offs in health care facility codes that can result in dramatic differences in construction costs. A major one is the use of sprinkler systems, for which costs can be reduced from $10 to $15 per square foot to approximately $2.50 per square foot for equivalent fire protection, while producing a building as safe as one meeting basic requirements.

The public has come to expect quality health care in buildings they have been led to believe are safe. That expectation does not come freely: it costs money to achieve desired levels of safety. And it is not necessary to have a major fire or structural failure to prove the point. Health care facility activities, by their very nature, place patients at risk medically (there are risks associated with many medical treatments, such as unconsciousness, drug reactions) as well as at risk physically (i.e., many patients would not be able to leave on their own because of the medical treatment they are receiving). To compensate for this, code requirements are more stringent, and thus more costly, for health care facilities. But to do less would be to jeopardize the safety of not only patients but also the staff, whose primary mission is the safety and welfare of patients entrusted to their care, and who therefore must remain with their patients under all circumstances.

CLASSIFYING CODES

The codes associated with building or renovating health care facilities can be divided into two major groups: those strictly related to the structure (facility codes) and those related to activities once the structure is built (operational codes).[3] Facility codes directly affect the process of building a facility. Operational codes also affect the building process, though not as obviously. As with any classification scheme, some codes contain requirements involving both groups.

Facility Codes

Today, facility codes are utilized during every aspect of building or renovating a structure. The following are the ones most related to health care facility projects.

Land Codes. Before a structure can be built, land codes need to be identified. These codes govern the use of the land and what is allowed to be built on a particular parcel. As might be expected, they differ from locality to locality. Codes in this category include zoning and environmental regulations.

Examples of *zoning regulations* are setback requirements, water and sewer drainage, curbing, and traffic movement (which, in most cases, are enforced by local and state authorities). *Environmental regulations* include wetland restrictions, pollution control, and earthquake considerations (which, in most cases, are handled by state and federal authorities).

Building Codes. These are the generic codes that cover general construction, and they include such items as structural integrity, material requirements, and heating, ventilation, and air conditioning (HVAC). These codes are necessary for erecting a physically sound structure. Codes in this category include the three model building codes[4] (basic building code, standard building code, and uniform building code); state building codes, which are sometimes one of the three model building codes adopted by reference and sometimes the state's own version; city building codes, which are again sometimes one of three model building codes adopted by reference and sometimes the city's own version; handicapped codes at the state and federal levels, which are requirements that must be met so that physically, visually, or audibly impaired persons can enter and travel within a building relatively unassisted; and U.S. Department of Health and Human Services *Guidelines for Construction and Equipment of Hospitals and Medical Facilities.*

> **NOTE:** These are guidelines unless adopted as a code by the state in which the project is located.

As might be expected, problems can arise if a state adopts one edition of a code and a local municipality another edition. The general rule in these instances is that the more restrictive requirement will prevail. However, owners should not hesitate to press for use of the less stringent edition if it is also the newer edition. A newer edition of a document reflects more research, reasoning, debate, technology, and other information, and if requirements have been relaxed, it only means that the old edition had been too conservative or promulgated without the benefit of additional research.

Fire Codes. Facility fire safety codes[5] have been developed over the years to meet the fire and explosion hazards that exist because of the way this planet functions: combustibles will burn in air given an ignition source. Fire codes set standards that attempt to prevent fires from occurring, suppress fires if they do start, or minimize the extent of damage until fire fighters arrive to extinguish the fire. Today, fire safety codes address the entire spectrum of building fire hazards: demolition and construction guidelines; building design as it relates to the ability to leave (or in some instances, particularly health care facilities, remain in) a building during a fire emergency; and operational practices as they affect building design.

Codes in these categories include the fire safety aspects of the following:

- Location of the structure with respect to adjacent buildings —that is, the fire exposure hazard both of the health care facility presenting a hazard to other buildings if it should burn, and of an adjacent building presenting a hazard to the health care facility if it should burn

- Area around the building—for example, storage facilities (gases, liquids, material, waste), parking garages, water supplies for fire-fighting purposes (hydrants, tanks), fire lanes, incinerators, and compactors

- Structural protection—for example, lightning protection, general construction protection, flame spread criteria of finish material, occupancy separation, windows and doors, laboratory construction criteria, chimney and fireplace criteria, floor and ceiling assemblies

- Life safety considerations—for example, adequate means of exiting; appropriate and adequate compartmentation of building; emergency lighting; appropriate fire protection systems for various occupancies; smoke control; additional protection for hazardous materials or areas

- Detection and extinguishment systems—for example, sprinkler systems, smoke, fire, and heat detector systems, fire pumps, standpipes, fire hoses

- Fixed building-wide service systems—for example, fuels and heating systems; air movement and restriction systems; electrical service (both normal and emergency); chutes for waste, linen, and other material, elevators; piped gas and vacuum systems

- Fixed localized systems—for example, storage areas (for gases, liquids, material, waste), computer centers, hyperbaric chambers, kitchen cooking equipment

It should be noted that building and fire codes sometimes cover the same subject in their respective documents, but for different purposes (e.g., fireproofing steel; material for doors; floor construction). Building codes are meant to protect buildings; fire codes are meant to protect people. These differences are sometimes forgotten or intermingled. Of late, there is a coordinated effort between the National Fire Protection Association and the model building codes groups to voluntarily coordinate requirements common to each so that they do not conflict with each other.

Mechanical Codes. The last major group of facility codes can be termed mechanical codes. Usually locally generated, they are generally associated with the trades and involve services within the building (see also Chapter 14 for the section on permits). Examples of what these codes cover are HVAC, plumbing, elevators, fuel location, lighting levels, and electricity.

Operational Codes

Operational codes are more difficult to take into account than facility codes when designing a health care facility because they are generally intended to be utilized by health care staff as they go about the business of caring for patients, as well as by architects and engineers as they design a building. Considering these codes means considering in advance of construction how people will function in the provision of health care services (both medical and nonmedical aspects). With the facility codes, the "object" (of the requirement) is not only known, but its location and movement (if any) are very predictable. With operational codes, the dimension of human operating needs and behavior must be added, and this makes matters much more complex.

Operational codes do not generally address the issue of design

and how requirements may affect it. However, their requirements do affect design. The following are a few examples:

1. Since essential electrical systems are necessary, the size of
   the emergency generator depends on what is to be connected to the generator in an emergency; this, in turn, affects the size of the room or area in which the generator will
   be housed.

2. The use of flammable anesthetics requires additional items
   to be installed in an anesthetizing location.[6]

3. The amount of flammable and combustible liquids and gases
   on site will affect the storage requirements for these
   products.

4. Areas that will be used as disaster control centers in an
   emergency need the capability and capacity for rapid
   expansion.

5. Will there ever be patients who are so infectious that an
   isolation room, and all that goes along with it, will be
   necessary?

6. If electronic equipment is to be maintained in-house, a
   space must be provided.

7. Will radioactive materials be used?

8. How are hazardous wastes to be disposed of?

Some issues are covered in fire codes, since they address the
protection of people. Other solutions are to be found in health
codes and regulations, which are concerned with the safety and
health of patients and staff. Others are contained in emergency
and civil defense regulations, which affect those facilities designated as emergency shelters. Still others are addressed by the
Occupational Safety and Health Administration (OSHA).

IMPACT OF CODES ON DESIGN

There is no question that codes, like nature, politics, or community opinion, place certain restrictions on structural aspects of
design (e.g., column diameters, the number of fire separations on
a floor, the extent of smoke compartmentation, the type and
extent of exterior glass). A skillful designer, however, can use the

codes to his or her advantage, with some forethought. A sprinkler system, for example, can be installed such that only flush-mounted caps are visible. A rated 2-hour door does not look much different from a rated 1-hour door.[7] Receptacles on essential power circuits need only be a different color to distinguish them from receptacles on normal power circuits.

Codes are developed as a response to some condition or event. Designers must therefore respond in kind by learning how to use the codes and not look at them as obstacles. If codes pertinent to a project are used from the beginning, a functionally aesthetic building is quite possible and will still be within the bounds of the codes.

NOTES

1. The term *code* as used in this book refers to the entire spectrum of documents developed for the purposes described in this chapter, whether voluntarily used or regulatory enforced.

2. For a scholarly treatment on the development of codes in the private sector, see R. G. Dixon, Jr., *Standards Development in the Private Sector: Thoughts on Interests, Representation and Procedural Fairness.* National Fire Protection Association, 1978.

3. There are efficacy codes that relate to the need for judging how well a product is doing what it is designed to do — for example, a pacemaker putting out the correct pulses; a scale measuring the weights it is designed for. However, these types of codes are not discussed here.

4. The model building codes refer to three voluntary, nongovernment groups that each produce a building code. They are the Building Officials and Codes Administrators International, whose document is titled the Basic Building Code; the International Conference of Building Officials, whose document is titled the Uniform Building Code; and the Southern Building Officials Congress International, whose document is titled the Standard Building Code. As the groups' names imply, each comprises government building officials and code enforcers (e.g., building department inspectors, fire marshals). Further, when each group revises its document, voting is restricted to government building officials and enforcers who have paid dues. Anyone, however, can submit recommendations to change these codes.

These three groups' codes are referred to collectively as the model building codes because their codes serve as models for states and municipalities, which often adopt one of the codes (either in whole or by reference). Like many developers of voluntary standards, these three groups can only recommend that their documents be adopted and enforced as written.

Over the years, three regions of the United States have each come to favor a specific code: the Northeast and Midwest primarily use the Basic Building Code; the Midwest and West, the Uniform Building Code; and the South, the Standard Building Code. Because these boundaries are not absolute, it is necessary to check with local and state building departments to learn which model building code is being used in the area, if at all.

5. See Appendix D, Health Care Firesafety Compendium, 1987, for a detailed listing of fire safety – related documents.

6. Flammable anesthetics are now used only rarely in the United States. However, the frequency of use does impact on the application of code requirements if flammable anesthestics are going to be used. Thus, the codes are very explicit in having facilities indicate whether an anesthetizing location is designated for the use of flammable anesthetics.

7. A rated fire door is a door constructed to resist fire and heat for a designated period of time.

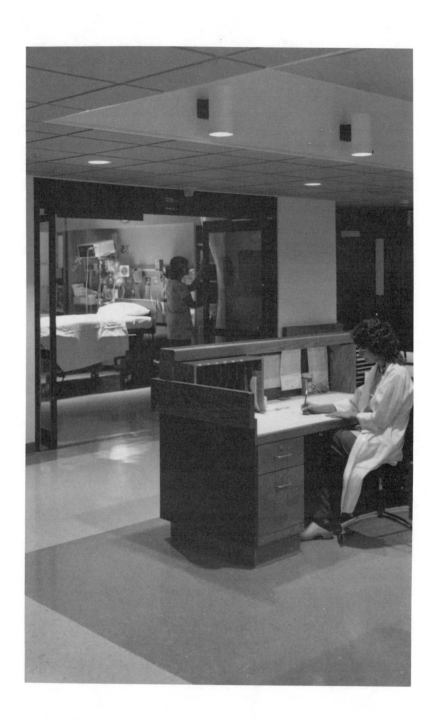

Part III

Construction and Beyond

CHAPTER 12

Drawings

Even the simplest renovation of or addition to a health care facility requires drawings indicating specifically and exactly what is to be built and where.[1] The drawing phase is difficult because it is the time that ideas and perceptions are translated into lines on paper (either as pictures or as words). Individuals such as the contractor need those lines to convert the ideas into physical structures. During that process, it may seem that the technical aspects (e.g., casework drawings, plans) have little connection to those original ideas. Be assured, however, that there is a definite connection between the concepts and a set of drawings that describes what is to be built.

It is also through the development of drawings that firm and reasonably accurate cost estimates can be established since the drawings provide the data for actual construction.

WHEN ARE DRAWINGS STARTED? (SKETCH STAGE)

Interestingly enough, drawings start with sketches formulated in the minds of the owners. If the owner, or his or her staff, has a technical background, or has studied drafting, these mind sketches can be drawn in rough form for presentation at interview meetings with prospective architects (see Chapter 7 on selecting the architect). These initial sketches can be developed long before any formal plans for building are readied.

When an architect does become involved with a project, he or she will develop a series of sketches that depict various professional solutions that are possible to implement the ideas of the owner or address the results of the evaluations discussed in Chapter 8. This is the architect's "homework" phase, when he or she will be starting the process of translating desires and dreams into real designs. Programs and studies will now be reviewed in great depth, with space and functioning aspects reduced to lines on paper. After the owner's initial approval of all the architect's ideas, a composite of the results can be generated in the form of scale drawings. These are usually done on a scale with $\frac{1}{16}$ inch representing 1 actual foot (generally shown or referred to as $\frac{1}{16}$-inch scale). For new facilities, this will determine the medical, supportive, and administrative activities able to take place in the new building or buildings as well as the space necessary for mechanical systems (e.g., boilers, air conditioning), storage areas, stairs, vents, and structural members. For existing facilities, this will determine how much of an area must be renovated in order to meet the changes desired. Scale drawings will also allow an initial check for code compliance, an initial review by pertinent health care agencies, and an initial cost analysis.

> **NOTE:** By this time, site and subsoil data will be necessary. See Chapter 5 for details.

If Certificate of Need (CON) approval is in process, these initial scale drawings will be necessary as accompaniment to the financial feasibility statement, which in turn will be part of the presentation to the CON board.

> **WARNING:** The requirements of the CON board in the state where work is to be done must be determined. Each state has slightly differing requirements. For example, some states require submission of alternative designs in order to see which is most cost-effective; some states require $\frac{1}{16}$-inch scale drawings, others $\frac{1}{8}$-inch scale drawings.

MORE AND MORE DETAILS (BASIC SCALE STAGE)

Following initial scale drawings, design development drawings, or basic scale drawings, are generated. These drawings are usually of $\frac{1}{8}$-inch scale and involve, as appropriate, plans of the building, elevations, and site work. (The last item refers again to Chapter 5.)

At this time, engineering assistance is necessary to advise on space requirements for heating, ventilation, and air conditioning

(HVAC) items and utility restrictions and availability. The persons who do this type of work are called structural, HVAC, plumbing, and electrical engineers.

Since even these drawings have limits on the information they can convey, as even more information will be necessary in order for construction to occur, a specification book is generally started about this time. The specification book describes the parts of the project in a detailed, technical way that would otherwise make drawings very cluttered or difficult to follow, particularly in the descriptions of how to do a particular procedure. There are specialists called specification writers who prepare specification books so that architects, engineers, tradespeople, enforcers, and others can understand what is desired or needed. Careful correlation with drawings is essential in preparing the specification book.

A CONSTANT LOOK AT COSTS

As mentioned, drawings provide a reference to review costs. At the sketch level, general estimates are possible. For more accurate costing, more detailed drawings must be developed.

At the basic scale drawing period, a review with owners should be conducted at least several times. These reviews are necessary because the drawings by this time will be very detailed and will allow very good cost estimates to be generated. The level of detail of the drawings and the reviews will also allow the cost capability of the facility to be factored into the final set of drawings and into the way the area or building will actually be built (i.e., which plan is possible?). CON board requirements, relative to costs, must also be learned during this period of cost estimating (i.e., can the facility spend X amount of dollars?). Otherwise, redrawing, and thus additional costs, may be necessary if the CON board approves a different dollar amount than anticipated.

WHO ACTUALLY DOES THE DRAWINGS?

Drawings are made by various people. In many cases, the architect does the concept drawings. In small offices, architects may also do the actual hard-line work. However, most drawings are made by skilled drafters. They use equipment as ancient as the pen and straight edge and as modern as computers to generate drawings. Techniques now available allow them to produce multicolor, shaded, and superimposed drawings. Drafters are supervised by a project coordinator, who in most instances has risen through the administrative ranks and has acquired the experience to coordinate the many pieces that compose a set of drawings.

The final set of drawings for a project are made on fine-grade drafting paper, mylar plastic, or cloth with ink or pencil. Because many copies of the set of drawings will be needed, drawings are printed by a process that results in so-called blue-line or black-line prints on a white background.[2]

Throughout the drawing period, drawings are constantly checked and rechecked by the architect and responsible engineer to make sure that all the work involved in the project is included either on the drawings or in the specification book. If something is left out at this stage, it can be a very costly error, in time and money, to correct after construction has commenced.

As mentioned in Chapter 7, computers are being used to generate drawings as the technology becomes more sophisticated and enables the storage and access of larger quantities of data. (The software is called computer-aided design.) For automating drawings, the storage of many equations and reference data tables is needed. More and more, the drafter is setting aside the pencil, the straight edge, and a large set of reference books for a computer terminal and an automated data retrieval system.

NEW FORMS OF DRAWINGS

Another exciting departure from the way the contents of drawings are drawn and displayed is provided by the mylar overlay system. Conventional drawings place everything, or nearly everything, for an area (such as an entire floor or room) on one sheet. With the mylar overlay system, the various systems for the same area (e.g., ductwork, steam, electrical low tension, electrical power, fire alarms, sprinklers) are each placed on a separate mylar print. The systems line up, when placed on top of each other, because the skeleton of the building or area is first generated on each mylar print and holes are punched out along the edges, directly beneath each other on every sheet. Thus, as prints are placed on top of each other, the systems will appear as they would if only one drawing were made of all the systems.

Although the cost per sheet is currently more expensive than that of conventional drawings, the advantages of the mylar overlay system are impressive:

1. Each system can be tracked more easily (e.g., each system can be drawn in different colors).

2. Areas where space is tight can be seen very quickly.

3. Drawings (prints) can be projected onto a screen very easily.

4. Contractors can study and follow each system separately or in groups.

5. Renovation work is eased as the method identifies work as it actually was done in any particular system.

6. Storage requirements of computer-generated drawings are simplified since only one system's data will have to be accessible at any one time.

7. Although there are more drawings for a project, each drawing is much simpler in detail and thus easier to understand.

8. The accuracy of costing out a project is increased.

9. The owner, in particular the facility engineer, benefits after completion of the project, since all systems require maintenance or repair at sometime, and the location and routing of each will be easier.

This method is beginning to grow in use and could become the general way of generating drawings within the next 5 to 10 years.

THE FINAL, APPROVED SET OF DRAWINGS (WORKING DRAWING STAGE)

While drawings are going through various iterations, the final details for a new structure or renovation have to be determined for incorporation into the working drawings and specification book.

It is at this time that the working drawings and specifications are done. They are generally drawn at a $\frac{1}{8}$-inch scale, with special areas enlarged to $\frac{1}{4}$-inch scale or even larger, if necessary. These drawings represent what is actually to be built. When completed, they are considered ready for:

1. Final approval by the owner
2. Final approval by enforcement agencies (e.g., CON board, state health department, state fire marshal, local building department
3. Submission for bid in order to obtain a price to carry out the project (i.e., construction)
4. Final cost estimate

> **NOTE:** A complete coordination with all involved trades is required at this stage as well.

If a construction management method or similar approach to construction is used, then a price for construction can be obtained when basic scale drawings[3] are completed. The price so obtained may be guaranteed by the contractor and/or may be subject to review and revision when final working drawings are completed. (See Chapter 14 for details on why this method is sometimes used.)

> **WARNING:** Whatever method of construction is selected, if a preset price is determined, there should be careful supervision during the working drawing stage so as not to increase the price of items, space, or equipment not fully accounted for at the time of the price guarantee. This is the most common area for disagreement as a project proceeds. It can result in dissatisfied owners, which in turn can lead to lawsuits that create undesirable feelings at all levels and on all sides.

TYPES OF WORKING DRAWINGS

The drawings described thus far have been discussed in the context of time — that is, when they are generated. The following are the different types of drawings that can be necessary, depending on the extensiveness of the project. Whereas all health care facility owners and staff may not need to know how to read these drawings, it behooves them to have some understanding of those portions of the project (and hence drawings) that affect them. This includes not only technical staff, such as facility engineers, but also medical and nursing staff. As examples, surgeons should know about the air-changing characteristics that will be used in operating rooms; nurses should know how much bed space per patient is being planned in intensive care units, medical and surgical patient rooms; laboratory workers should know how air will be drawn up fume hoods; and security and risk managers should know how the alarm systems will operate. This information will all be explained graphically and verbally in drawings and the specification book. The various types of drawings and their components are described as follows.

Title sheet. This indicates the building(s) and the location(s), the owner, the architect or engineer, and the date. Some states or agencies require the seal of an architect or engineer on the title sheet. If this is the case, space should be blocked out for seals or stamps of the architect or engineer and any required agencies.

Abbreviations, indexes, general notes, and miscellaneous data. This information is just that.

Site survey. This is completed by a surveyor with a registered seal who has been hired by the owner to survey the required land area. Identification of the surveyor is required.

Subsoil data. This is a record of subsoil information that has been completed by a competent company hired by the owner. Identification of an authorized representative of the company is required.

Site plan. This indicates new or revised work to be done on the site. The plan is created by the architect or a registered landscape architect or a civil engineer. It should indicate all details appropriate to the work: sections of the grading, light pole details, patios, roads, curbs, curb cuts, handicapped requirements, ramps, steps, flag poles, walks, parking layouts, drainage, hydrants, and site utilities.

NOTE: If extensive road or regrading is required, a civil engineer should be consulted.

Planting plan. This drawing indicates all planting and landscape decoration and identifies all trees, shrubs, and plantings by name and size. It should by means of the specification book indicate planting procedures, fertilizers to be used, and proper care. Details for tree support and special items such as benches, fountains, and special effects should be included as necessary.

Existing building(s) (demolition plan). This drawing indicates the extent of all areas to be demolished or to remain. This plan must therefore be very clear so that the starting point for construction (i.e., the new project) is the way the contractor expects it. Particular attention must be paid to the type of existing partitions, equipment, piping, ductwork, insulation, asbestos, stairs, shafts, elevators, dumbwaiters, and roofing. Use of descriptive notes is encouraged to explain intent in full. There should also be a note indicating who is to retain the salvage (owner or contractor) and/or how it is to be disposed of. A separate plan for each floor or area is required.

Existing building(s) (elevation). This is another drawing relative to work to be done to existing structures. Items of consideration here include window replacement, caulking, brick repair or cleaning, gutters, roofing, and painting.

Floor plans (new or alterations). These drawings indicate all new areas or areas to remain. It includes room names, dimensions, door swing, smoke partitions, and fire partitions.

> **NOTE:** Some architectural offices devise methods to show door sizes, types, dimensions, and material on separate sheets to facilitate the totaling of the number of doors needed. This is acceptable if it does not make it difficult to follow drawings.

A floor plan of *each* floor must be drawn. One sheet with a note that it represents several identical floors can be confusing and create problems (e.g., the numbering for rooms).

Elevations (new or alterations). These drawings are a view of all new areas or areas to remain. It includes the materials, dimensions, window locations, doors, canopies, and all features required to complete the desired architectural complex (i.e., complementing the floor plan). It also indicates a true ground-to-building relationship, such as the way the ground slopes or an uneven line unless the ground next to the building is perfectly horizontal. It should also show all expansion and/or construction joints; all code requirements, such as tempered or wired glass; and any retention screens, louvers, rails, or window cleaning equipment. Elevation drawings are required for all sides, that is, a frontal view for every wall.

> **WARNING:** Items that do *not* enhance the aesthetic appearance of the drawing are to be included. Eleva-

tions are not intended to be perspective drawings or paintings. Pipes show as pipes where pipes are and so do louvers.

Wall sections and details. This indicates typical and/or special sections through exterior walls. They should also indicate exterior windows and door details. This may involve several sheets, depending on the complexity and size of the project. Repeating entire typical sections to show a particular special section should be avoided.

Interior details. Interior door schedules, interior windows ("borrowed light"), interior partition details, benches, supports, corner guards, handrails, bumpers, and other items pertinent to a particular project are shown.

Reflected ceiling plans. This drawing of the ceiling indicates material, grid layout, light locations, smoke detectors, sprinkler head locations, vents, speakers, curtain rails, intravenous tracks, soffits, and other ceiling features pertinent to a particular project. A reflected ceiling plan is required for each floor.

Casework. Casework is built-in cabinetry, both floor mounted and wall or ceiling hung. This drawing indicates plans and details of all casework involved in a project.

Special details. All details for special areas associated with a project are drawn. These include chapels, coffee shops, gift shops, lobbies, lounges, boardrooms, laundries, sterilizing rooms, radiology rooms, operating rooms, and patient rooms. In most cases, these drawings require floor plans on a larger scale for detail purposes.

Room finish schedule and color material layouts (including furniture layouts). Final detail work for each room is represented.

> **NOTE:** Some architectural offices split these items into separate sheets to allow easier reading of each on the project. The combination of room finish and color may in some cases become too cumbersome to include on just one sheet. Room finish and color can also be included in the specification book.

Fire and safety plans. Some states (e.g., Florida) require a separate plan for each floor devoted to fire and safety requirements, such as location of fire hose cabinets, smoke detectors, sprinklers, and exit signs.

HVAC site plan. All exterior work for HVAC (e.g., steam lines) is drawn.

HVAC floor plan (demolition). This drawing indicates all existing areas to be demolished or retained. As noted for demolition of existing buildings, disposal of salvage must be indicated.

HVAC floor plans. This drawing indicates all work to be completed for ductwork and pertinent equipment (including dampers) and piping and pertinent equipment, with each on separate sheets.

HVAC details. All required details for completion of this work are shown.

> **WARNING:** It must be noted who furnishes and details exterior louvers to avoid a disagreement between the architect and HVAC engineer over what type is used.

HVAC riser diagrams. This drawing indicates all riser diagrams needed to install HVAC equipment.[4]

Plumbing site work. All exterior plumbing work must be depicted. This includes such items as all connections to utilities, catch basins, manholes, hydrants, and drain inlets. In this regard, rainfall, runoff data, and water table level data may be required. Information on water pressure for domestic, fire riser, and sprinkler operation is required.

> **NOTE:** The required pressure at the top of the system can be obtained from local authorities.

Plumbing floor plans (demolition). This drawing shows all items to be removed or retained. Again, disposition of salvage must be indicated. A plan for each floor is required.

Plumbing floor plans. All new or retained plumbing work, including the types of fixtures, is shown. A plan for each floor is required.

Plumbing floor plan (sprinklers). All sprinklers and pertinent equipment, including fire pumps, and fire risers, are drawn. A plan is required for each floor. This drawing may have to be approved by a state sprinkler agency. Again, water pressure for the system can be obtained from local authorities.

Plumbing riser diagrams. All riser diagrams required to complete the project are indicated.

Plumbing details. All details required for the project are shown.

NOTE: Piped gas systems (medical and nonmedical) are designed by the plumbing engineer. Thus, a drawing of the floor plan showing each piped gas system must be included.

Electrical site plan. This drawing indicates all exterior electrical work, such as at entrances, for connections to utilities, and parking lighting.

Electrical floor plans (demolition). This shows all areas to be demolished or retained. Again, disposal of salvage must be noted.

Electrical floor plans. Here, there will be at least several drawings covering the following systems: floor plans — power and light, which could be on separate sheets, and floor plans — low tension, which could be divided into communications and other systems. These drawings must show all items and equipment required to complete the project.

Electrical details. This drawing indicates all electrical details, such as lights by type, wiring for items, floor-run ductwork, conduits and raceways, and special requirements. Coordination with the electrical floor plan (previous drawing) is essential.

Electrical riser diagrams. This drawing shows all required riser diagrams, all transfer switches to emergency power generator equipment, and connections to all dampers and other mechanical equipment.

Special drawings. These are done as needed. They include:

- Asbestos removal. Drawings are needed if reinsulating for equipment, piping, or ductwork is required. A check with state and federal requirements is advised because of environmental impact.

- Radiation protection. If equipment utilizing radioactive materials is used, drawings are required by departments of radiology of state health departments to include such items as protection (i.e., lead) diagrams.

- Radio frequency (rf) interference. Drawings indicate how protection from elevators and other sources is to be achieved for electrocardiographic and similar equipment that is sensitive to magnetic fields generated by large motors when they start.

Shop drawings (details). During construction of a project, the manufacturers and fabricators of certain items prepare drawings, brochures, or written specifications to ensure their equipment is installed correctly. It is the responsibility of the architect and engineer to review these drawings for compatibility with the project. The contractor must also review and sign them. Any substitutions must be noted, with the reasons given and the owner so advised.

Detailed drawings. During construction, the architect or engineer may be required to provide detailed drawings of explanation to facilitate the work of the contractor. These drawings are not of changes and thus are not change orders. Rather, they are generated to explain a very complicated, and possibly confusing, situation such as how a particular piece of equipment fits into a certain space.

THE CHANGE-ORDER DRAWING

Another category of drawings that is least desired by all parties is the change-order drawing. It represents problems beyond those to be generally expected when building according to the approved set of drawings. Unless the change is a significant reduction in the total project, a change-order drawing will involve cost and time, both of which must be justified. These drawings can become necessary for several reasons, such as:

1. Someone changes his or her mind.

2. The original material specified is no longer available.

3. The subsoil data was not 100% percent accurate.

4. A different configuration is necessary or desired after bid.

Sometimes these changes require only a little extra work; sometimes they require a lot of extra work. Similarly, material costs can increase or decrease because of the change. The reason or fault, if any, for the change must be determined, and any cost differences agreed on before the change can be accomplished.

For purposes of this chapter, a drawing and/or a written description detailing the change order must be generated and then signed by the owner, the architect and engineer, and the contractor. All this—the change, the drawing reflecting the change, and the sign-off—must be accomplished before any work associated with the change is started. (See Chapter 14 for more details on these types of changes.)

AS-BUILT DRAWINGS

The as-built drawings, which show the final way that construction was completed, are discussed in Chapter 16.

NOTES

1. There are many types of drawings, and more than one name is used by different persons for a particular type of drawing. The terms used in this book are the ones we have used or heard used most often.

2. In the past, drawings were made on fine-grade linen. Today this is too costly. Also, before blue-line prints were developed, blueprints were used. This term was coined because the copying technique resulted in white line work on a blue background.

3. This term, although not the official one of the American Institute of Architects (AIA), is used often by many architectural and design offices. The AIA term is *design development drawings*.

4. A riser diagram is a vertical indication of pipes, ducts, or electrical lines.

CHAPTER 13

Ground Breaking

Is ground breaking a worthwhile tradition or an expensive publicity affair? We feel it is the former, and this chapter highlights some of the reasons why there are benefits to holding such an event, as well as details on how to plan and hold a ground-breaking ceremony.

One note of caution, however, is that if a ground-breaking ceremony is held, it should be carried out well, with nothing left to chance. A badly run ground-breaking ceremony can be a turn-off in many ways and can haunt a facility for years afterward.

WHY BOTHER?

There are no requirements or regulations that ground-breaking ceremonies be held. It is a matter of personal choice. The addition of a new loading dock area or the renovation of administrative offices does not stir the asking of whether a ground-breaking ceremony should be held. But a new patient wing, a new laboratory or patient building, or almost anything that requires a new foundation generally does raise the question of whether some kind of ceremonial first turn of earth should be held.

The genealogy of ground breaking is obscure. It is known that many elaborate ceremonies, including the sacrifice of humans, were held in ancient times at the rise of new temples to please the gods. In medieval times, human sacrifices disappeared, but the ceremony was retained.

Today ground breaking is a formal marker, indicating that the next stage in the building process is about to take place: actual construction. It is one time in the building cycle that owners can publicly call attention to the merits of the projects they have undertaken and thank supporters of the project. Ground break-ings have also become media events in some instances.

Because of this importance, a certain amount of orchestration of the ceremony is required to control events, and not have events control the ceremony. A ground-breaking event repre-sents another opportunity to foster goodwill with residents in the area and the public at large. Thus, a project that has involved so much work to reach this stage deserves some sort of ceremony.

PLANNING

As the building of a facility requires planning, so too does a ground breaking ceremony. This planning can start as early as when it is certain that construction will take place.

For continuity, one person should be designated as coordinator of the event. For an existing facility, this can be a member of administration, such as from a public affairs department. It could be a volunteer who has been active in the project and, more important, is experienced in planning public events. Or it could be a paid consultant, such as someone from a public relations firm. Whatever route is followed, a committee under the owner should be formed to handle all aspects of the ceremony and to work with any public relations firm that may be retained.

The major areas of concern in any ground-breaking ceremony are the invitation list, media coverage, logistics for the event, and orchestration of the ceremony.

Invitees

Invitations for these affairs can be a sensitive issue: who is not invited can be just as important as who is invited. A general rule is to invite if there is any question. But effort should be expended to learn of all groups that will be affected by the project and to invite either representatives of or the entire group itself.

The following list (not in order of priority) is provided to show how much thought should be given to the question of whom to invite. As with any function, appropriateness and common sense should prevail. Potential guests include:

- Members of any building committee

- Local groups—civic, religious, social, cultural, youth, health. They may have to use the facility eventually; they are also potential fund-raisers.

- Members of the local community. They will be affected by the structure if it happens to be a large one; it is good public relations to invite the public.

- Donators. It is good personally as well as morally to recognize those who have already donated money to the project.

- Elected officials — local (e.g., mayor), state (e.g., area representatives), even federal (e.g., district representatives, senators)

- Career government employees — local (e.g., fire department, police department), state (e.g., public health department), federal (e.g., Department of Health and Human Services)

- Architect and engineer. They need to feel involved; it will make for a stronger team.

- Contractor(s). *All* of those with whom a contract has been signed should be invited.

- Current employees. If the project is an addition, the ground breaking will be a good time to bring them up-to-date.

The Media

For media coverage, there are considerations before, during, and after the ceremony to consider. Today, media coverage is a necessity, although sometimes the media will come even without an invitation because the project has become news in some way.

Before the ceremony, an information sheet should be prepared that explains the purpose and extent of the project. It should include a diagram of the proposed structure or area, a brief description of the project, a summary of what will take place at the ceremony, who will be speaking, and who should be contacted for additional information. The media cannot be forced to cover the event; they can only be asked. It is important, therefore, that the information sheet be sufficiently detailed for the media to judge fairly whether to cover the event. It should also be attractive.

A list of media in the area should thus be drawn up during this time. It should include all local daily and weekly newspapers, all trade journals, and all local radio and television stations. The information sheet should be mailed out in advance of the ceremony — at least several weeks prior to the day. If 6 to 8 weeks' notice can be given, then a follow-up letter or call can be made about 3 weeks before the event to those who have not responded; this will also help establish a more personal relationship with the media.

During the ceremony, a media contact, preferably the same contact listed in the information sheet, should be present to answer questions about what will take place, how long speakers will talk, where cameras can best be placed, and other concerns. Members of the media, for their part, will be asking for group pictures before the ceremony and for candid pictures during the ceremony. They may also want to interview key persons involved in the project before the ceremony. However, owners and staff should not be surprised if media members leave before the end of events. They may have deadlines to meet or other events to cover.

One note of caution is that if there has been any public controversy along the way over the project, one can be sure the media will be present and ask about the situation. Problems today that can cause public reaction include pollution, traffic congestion, neighborhood intrusion or destruction, and types of proposed services or research. Problems can sometimes be opportunities, and a ground-breaking ceremony can be a time to state the facility's side of an issue. Owners and administrators should not be reluctant to point out the benefits they see from the proposed project.

After the ceremony, periodic progress reports to the media can be helpful to keep them informed of what is happening on the project. They help retain media interest should a dedication ceremony be held (see Chapter 16) and may serve to prevent a distant or even hostile relationship from developing.

Logistics for the Day

A ground-breaking ceremony can be as simple or expansive as desired. Whatever is done, a certain amount of logistics must be considered in order to have an orderly event. These include:

1. Date and time of ceremony. A check of other events that have already been scheduled for that day could be a worthwhile exercise.

2. Backup plan for poor weather. Since the ceremonial turning of earth will be outdoors, provisions for inclement weather should be considered. Adequate space should be set aside to prevent crowding.

3. To stand or sit? This will depend on how long the ceremony will last and how many people are expected. A short ceremony is preferable to a long one; it is also preferable to have seating when available. With an existing building, part of the ceremony could be held in the existing structure if seating is available there.

4. Reception. Hosting a reception will depend on whether the project is a new wing and there is an existing structure that can be used; whether there is any space to hold a reception; or whether conditions at the site deem that a reception can be held there. Any reception should be within walking distance of the ceremony. A formal dinner is not necessary or even desirable. Light refreshments (punch, pastries, perhaps wine are satisfactory.

5. Parking. Unless everyone has to come by public transportation, which is very unlikely, designation of parking areas should be very clear, with lanes left for emergency vehicles in case a sudden illness prompts the need for ambulance access. Cars should be parked in orderly rows: everyone trying to leave from randomly parked cars could result in no one being able to leave. Hence, there should be someone directing the parking as well as the exiting of cars.

The Ceremony

There are no specific rules on the way ground-breaking ceremonies have to be held. Aside from the traditional overturning of a spade or two of earth to symbolize that construction is beginning, almost anything can be done. There can be speeches, prayers, balloon launches, firing of cannons, sky writing, the overturning of many spades of earth, or the scooping out of a giant spade of earth by a bulldozer. Within reason, the more imaginative, the better.

At minimum, the owner or administrator should state the purpose of the project, when it was started, when it will be completed, and what benefit it will provide the community. It should not be assumed everyone will be familiar with the project.

No matter how long or short the ceremony will be, a program should be printed listing ceremony participants, their affiliation, and a brief description of the project, such as why it was started, who will benefit from it, and when it will be completed. A sketch of the completed structure is always in order. Such a program will help latecomers as well as answer basic questions. It is also a tangible token of the event so that people do not have to just rely on memory.

There are a few final points. One person should be in charge of the ceremony, and it should be evident that he or she is the person in charge. Any sound system should be adequate for the size of the audience anticipated as well as the ambient noise level that may exist. Finally, the media's need for pictures and interviews should not be hampered. Group shots before the ceremony and candid shots during the ceremony should be discussed in advance.

A final caution is that the unexpected is always possible, no matter how much planning is done. If problems do arise, it is unwise to overreact to them. Acknowledging and accepting the problems will be viewed as more mature than creating an embarrassing scene.

CHAPTER 14

The Construction Process

The many facets of the construction process, from obtaining permits to having inspections done, are the subject of this chapter.

PERMITS

Permits, or permission to build, are another checkpoint by local governments to help ensure that whatever is built within their jurisdiction is done according to established rules and regulations. Permits are another part of a government's responsibility to protect its citizenry: in this instance, against poorly built structures that would pose structural as well as fire hazards. They are the way quality assurance is achieved for the general public, assuming there are honest, responsible government officials. Permits allow public officials to monitor construction of a structure and to take action to correct any deficiencies that would endanger occupants or visitors in the structure.

Who Obtains Them?

Generally, the contractor is required to obtain the various permits needed to build or renovate a structure. Subcontractors may also be required to obtain subpermits. (See the subsequent section for an abridged list of the types of permits associated with health care facility projects.)

Once obtained, permits should be conspicuously displayed to save unnecessary time looking for them if questions arise.

Who Issues Them?

Generally, the local building inspector in the building department either issues all the permits that are necessary or coordinates their issuance with other departments or agencies, such as the electrical department, fire department, or public safety department. Before issuing permits, a building inspector also requires that all zoning and any bylaws of the jurisdiction be cleared. Proof of Certificate of Need (CON) approval is necessary when applying for these permits.

These departments and inspectors have specific roles throughout the construction process. Department personnel review building plans for compliance to regulations adopted within their jurisdiction (e.g., building, fire safety, health). During construction, they also make inspections of such items as foundation integrity, weldings, and wiring since these and other related items would be enclosed (hidden) after construction is completed. Inspectors also make final checks of a structure to ensure that everything in general, with respect to safety regulations, has been complied with. (Interim and final inspections and approvals are discussed in detail later in this chapter and in Chapter 15.)

Types of Permits

Permits are trade related; that is, they cover many of the trades that are necessary to erect a building or renovate an area. Depending on the extensiveness of the project and the regulations that a jurisdiction has adopted, any or all of the following permits might be necessary before construction could begin:

1. General building permit — issued, for example, when any structural changes are made; when load-bearing walls are modified; when an entire building is being erected

2. Foundation permit — issued, for example, when pile driving is done, caissons used, or footings poured

3. Crane operation permit — issued, for example, when steel girders have to be hoisted and a crane is required

4. Elevator permit — issued, for example, when a temporary elevator has to be assembled for hoisting material or personnel and when a permanent elevator is to be installed

5. Gas installation permit

6. Oil tank installation permit

7. Electrical wiring installation permit

8. Plumbing installation permit

9. Oil or gas-heating equipment permit

10. Heating, air conditioning, and ventilating permit

It is incumbent upon contractors to learn which permits are required by the jurisdiction in which the project is to be located.

Cost of Permits

Fees for permits range from nothing, to a nominal fee, to a percentage of the total construction cost and/or total square footage to be constructed (each floor of a multistory building is figured into that total square footage). The cost of permits also depends on whether the local or state government wants to charge whatever is necessary for the building department to be self-sufficient or whether part of the funds for operating the department is to come from general revenue (i.e., taxes). This issue, however, is beyond the scope of this book.

If a state requires a review of drawings prior to construction, some graduated fee is probable—that is, the larger the project, the larger the fee. In lieu of doing the review themselves (and thus charging for it), some states require a third party (not the architect/engineer of record) to review drawings and specifications prior to issuing a permit. This review is not free either.

> **NOTE:** The third party is a state-approved architect or engineer.

The classification of an institution is not a factor in permit costs. Nonprofit and religious institutions pay the same fee as do for-profit institutions.

Time Limitations on Permits

Similar to driver licenses and most credit cards, permits are valid for a specified time. But unlike these two items, a permit's validity relates to when work must *commence* on the project (in most cases, within 90 days of issuance).

> **NOTE:** CON boards also set a maximum time in which construction is to start; otherwise a facility must resubmit plans for approval. In addition, CON boards require quarterly reports on construction progress and costs incurred.

Government Requirements

In issuing permits, local, state, and federal governments have adopted procedures and regulations that must be followed by owners and contractors. These include advertising, bidding, non-discrimination, and minority group involvement. Each project is checked by authorized or designated local, state, and federal agencies for compliance against these requirements.

Thus, contractors have to do some careful and thorough time planning in order to have work commence as originally desired, and not spend time and money reapplying for new permits.

CONSTRUCTION METHODS

The decision as to which construction method should be used must be made long before ground breaking. In fact, discussions should be started at the time that financial matters are under review (see Chapter 3).

The six construction methods discussed subsequently are not unique to health care facility construction. They are just the ones most generally used. For the most part, health care facility construction projects are no different from other construction projects, though specific requirements for facilities themselves may differ significantly.

Whatever method is used, local, state, and federal regulations relative to antidiscrimination, small businesses, minority groups, insurance coverage, bonding, warranties, and work performance must be followed. The owner and contractor are both responsible for adhering to these policies.

Straight Bid Construction

This method is used when several qualified contractors are asked to bid on a project that has been put on the market after drawings and specifications have been approved. The list of contractors will vary depending on whether the project is financed by private money or public money. In most cases, a list of subcontracts for major portions of the work will be required to be submitted by the prime contractor. If public money is involved, a prior bidding for these sub-bids (e.g., heating, ventilation, and air conditioning [HVAC]; plumbing; electric; carpentry; ironwork) will have to be held, and the prime contractor will be required to use the qualified low bid. In the case of private money, the owner will select the firms and it is not mandatory for the owner to accept the low bid.

Cost-Plus Method

This method is used when the contractor is selected without going through the bid process but does agree to submit all costs involved as work progresses. In most cases, a base figure of 10 percent is added to the base cost as the contractor's profit. Hence, this type of construction must have good up-front work. Exact knowledge of costs ahead of time should be the goal.

> **CAUTION:** This method can become a runaway project, with costs that keep increasing, and it is advised only for *small* projects with well-known local contractors.

Fast-Track Method

This method is derived from the name attached to construction when one or several attempts are made to do a project faster than the normal procedure. It is used by construction management groups to start construction (having given a construction price on partially completed plans) before drawings and specifications have been completed. This method also allows the preordering of major items, such as steel, or long-time order items, such as hardware or special equipment.

This method was popular when the rate of inflation was high, as time was the enemy then. The only argument for it now (while a low rate of inflation continues) is that is *might* get the project completed sooner, and thus have income generated sooner. It has not been proved that this method gets a job done faster. A job will certainly not be done better using this method, as working with incomplete data causes only frustration, anger, and dissatisfaction.

Construction Management Method

This method brings a construction firm on board early in the process. Its purpose is the use of a consultant who has actual cost experience in the field in order to avoid overruns and underruns in construction costs. A fee is charged for this service.

In most cases, the construction firm involved remains throughout the project, with the construction manager giving a guaranteed price of construction and being allowed to build the project. The construction manager is expected to assume all responsibilities for the costs he or she guarantees. The project can also go to bid and another contractor can be allowed to do the building, with costs still monitored by the construction manager. The latter (bid process) does not happen too often, however.

Design/Build or Turnkey Method

This method is used to design and build a project as a package. One company will design and then build the addition or new structure. It can be likened to buying a car right off the lot: you get what is there; there is no choice of color or options. You might get a good product; you might get a lemon.

Owner-Build Method

This method best suits very small in-house projects. The owner acts as his or her own contractor and subcontracts parts of the projects or uses his or her own staff. This will save money in terms of the prime contractor's profit and overhead.

> **CAUTION:** It is strongly advised that owners carry an appropriate level of insurance when using this method since facilities do not carry construction insurance. In addition, a check with local unions should be made. Some building trades might strike the facility if non-union personnel are doing their trade.

Observations

The straight bid method is perhaps the most time proven of all the various methods used. There is less latitude for manipulating the construction to profit a particular contractor.

In most cases in recent years involving the popular fast-track, construction management, and design/build methods, no strong proof has arisen to indicate that these methods have greatly saved money or time.

MIDCOURSE CORRECTIONS

The subject of changes after a contract has been signed is the most often encountered and least desired problem of a project. It is a deviation from the approved set of drawings and specification book. In particular, a major change to any part of a project as complex as the building of a health care facility will cause untold aggravation, lost tempers, and unbelievable costs. Thus, changes need to be reviewed carefully, weighing the direct and indirect ramifications from implementing the change.

When Is a Change a Change?

On any project, minor changes are almost always expected and even anticipated: an overlooked item; an updated item; an obsolete item; a corner too rounded; a corner not rounded enough; a clearance width not adequate. Corrective action for these types of problems can be taken as it will not disrupt progress much and will cost little or no extra money at this time. It would even probably save money, since attempts to make correction later would be even more disruptive to work flow.

A major change, however, is something else.[1] Changes in this category should be thought out carefully because of their consequences. A thorough discussion might reveal possible alternatives or simpler solutions (i.e., can the problem be reduced to a minor change?).

Causes of major changes are several: poor or inadequate original estimates; a vital (costly) item somehow overlooked; unclear drawings; an error during initial construction. Whatever the cause, major changes can be categorized as architect/engineer error or omission; owner requested; contractor caused or requested (e.g., something done in disagreement with the contract; a request to do a certain part of the project using a different method or material); or supplier change or unavailability.

The extent of a problem, and the resultant proposed change, will determine who pays for whatever is finally done. It is thus necessary to establish responsibility where possible. This becomes difficult, if not impossible, when the supplier is involved.

It is cautioned, however, that professional judgment should be exercised for all changes. Not every change can be deemed an error; and attempts to assign costs for every minor infraction will be counterproductive and could eventually jeopardize the project.

Although careful and thorough planning before construction can project most costs and careful reviews and checks during construction can indicate if problems are developing, deviations are almost inevitable. But they should not exceed 2 or 3 percent of planned construction costs.

In summary, changes can be expected, but careful planning will reduce their impact.

Determining the Cost of a Change

When all parties have agreed on the necessity of a change, and on the best way to make the change with the least disruption, the contractor will be responsible for obtaining the cost estimate for the change. This estimate will be reviewed in turn by the architect and the financial watchdogs of the project (e.g., the bank providing the largest loan, a financial committee or consultant).

> **NOTE:** If the change is relatively small, that is, below a preset limit, a major review by financial persons may not be necessary. However, no change should be formally initiated without the written approval of the owner.

An owner can obtain other estimates if it is felt the contractor's estimate is not reasonable. However, a proposed change does not give the owner the right to have the work associated with change done by someone else without the written approval of the original contractor. Another contractor might be used, though it is rare, if the proposed change involves a special trade.

It's All in the Time!

When the need arises for a possible change can influence *whether* it is going to be done. The byword here is "the sooner the better," for time plays a major role in the decision-making process.

There are approximately three time zones related to changes:

1. Construction has yet to begin. This is obviously the best time to discover a problem and rectify it. At this time, a change will cause the least amount of extra work and money since nothing will have to be demolished or returned to a vendor.

   > **NOTE:** There may be some cancellation charges for equipment already ordered.

2. Construction has begun involving the item to be changed. This is the most costly time for a change since work associated with the change has to be stopped. This in turn could affect adjacent or subsequent work, with an entire area's work slowed down. This change requires the most careful review in order not to disrupt the entire project.

3. Construction has been completed. This time may be too late to make the change. The original contractor may not want to, or even be able to, return to this problem. The costs associated with the change may be grounds for reconsideration of the need to make the change. The change might jeopardize the scheduled completion date (and thus the scheduled opening date of the new facility or renovated area).

INSPECTIONS ALONG THE WAY

As work on a project takes place, various inspections for different purposes will also take place. These inspections can be grouped into several categories.

One category is almost rhetorical: is the area, or structure, being built according to the plans? For example, are the specifications being followed? Are the various items being installed in the correct sequence? Are all the materials being stored correctly? Are various areas of the building being made available to the facility in order not to interfere with good medical practice?

Another is a check on the quality of the workmanship for safety purposes. For example, what is the integrity of welds and flooring? Are water pipes tight? Has the heating system been checked for clean ducts, leaks, and proper air supply and exhaust? Has the humidity control been checked? Have the oxygen and gas systems been checked and labeled?

A third is a check that items, equipment, and systems have been installed correctly and are operating as intended. Equipment may not be all provided or installed by the contractor, and the clerk of the works has to ensure that it is coordinated with the rest of the building.

A fourth check is on the quality of workmanship for appearance (i.e., finishing work quality). It is the final appearance of any product that is seen, not what went into its construction. Thus, the final touch can make or spoil an otherwise well-built structure (e.g., a crooked piece of casework; a misaligned ceiling fixture).

There are also inspections for safety during construction. These cover, among other things, that the site is clean and that open elevator shafts are protected. Since construction of a major project without some injury is rare, safety of all persons (workers and visitors) is a constant concern. (There is more discussion of safety in the next section.)

There will more than likely be several agencies inspecting the same work for the same or different reasons. A partial list follows of who will be regularly checking or inspecting a project or will be coming by irregularly, announced and unannounced, to inspect a project.

Who's Checking?

Clerk of the Works. On any major project, an owner will hire, or designate from his or her staff, a person to inspect daily the work being done to determine if it is in accordance with the plans, drawings, and specification book. This person, called the clerk of the works (see Glossary for definition), must be qualified in the construction field in order to understand the mechanics involved in translating drawings, designs, and specifications into a finished product. This person reports his or her findings to the owner and the architect/engineer, who in turn reviews them for any problems. The architect/engineer will prepare recommendations as to how the owner should proceed on any problems.

Architect/Engineer. They inspect a project personally throughout construction in order to be satisfied that work is producing results as intended.

Project Manager. For large projects, or when several are in progress simultaneously, contractors and builders also employ someone to make sure each project is being carried out according to plans, drawings, and specifications.

Inspection Agencies or Organizations. A host of groups inspect health care projects from beginning to end (and after). It thus behooves all sides in a project to learn which groups can be expected: both when and how often, since the intervals of inspection vary within each locality and state.

Building Inspector. This is the local authority who will begin checking from the beginning (e.g., foundations; stock; structural framing integrity before walls are installed). This person also issues the certificate allowing actual occupancy (see Chapter 15).

Fire Inspector. This can be a person from the local fire department or from the state fire marshal's office (or both). In some states, fire safety inspections can occur at the drawing stage, which means approval for drawings must be secured even before construction (see Types of Working Drawings in Chapter 12). Fire safety inspections will also occur as fire protection features are installed.

Department of Public Safety of the State. This department, or its equivalent, can be a separate agency or exist within a building or fire department. Its inspections could thus duplicate all or portions of these other two departments' inspections if it is a separate agency.

Occupational Safety and Health Administration (OSHA). This federal agency can inspect a project, at the request of an employee, for the safety methods used during construction (see also next section).

Insurance Underwriter. Insurance companies are very concerned about the property they are or will be insuring. Thus, they may inspect a project on their own volition or at the request of the owner.

Joint Commission on Accreditation of Healthcare Organizations (JCAHO). This nongovernment accrediting organization generally inspects a project after it is completed, relying on a statement of construction form completed by owners to learn of details. For projects on existing facilities (i.e., renovations), JCAHO allows the use of a fire safety evaluation system (FSES) to show equivalency on certain items.

> **NOTE:** The fire safety evaluation system must be approved by the JCAHO prior to construction. Also, other agencies may also allow the use of FSES.

Specific Inspectors. Some systems or fixed equipment require separate inspections during and after installation. This is to ensure that they have been installed properly and thus do not present a hazard. These inspections may be conducted by the manufacturer, by utility companies, or by the installer. They are always witnessed by the owner and local authorities. Inspections in this category include boiler and heating systems, oil tank installations, elevators, emergency electric generator systems, fire and smoke detection systems, and extinguishing systems.

Maintaining Safety During Construction

Another concern during construction that will result in inspection is the safety of the persons in and around the job site. Depending on the type of project, responsibility for this safety will vary between the owner and the contractor. For a new structure, or for renovation of a structure in which no patient or staff activity is taking place, the contractor will be responsible for maintaining safe working conditions. For renovations of or additions to health care facilities that are already functioning, safety will be the joint responsibility of the owner and contractor.

A checklist has been prepared for guidance on safety during construction (see Appendix F). It lists the major areas of concern and what precautions and/or preventive measures should be considered.

In meeting their responsibilities, contractors need to be observant of OSHA regulations; state and local labor and industry rules; state bonding regulations; carrying sufficient insurance for construction, failure of work, fire, flooding, and other contingencies; and worker's compensation laws. Inspections can be expected for any and all of these five items.

Although labor strikes are always a possibility when unions are involved, this should not interfere with conducting business in a normal, professional manner. Good working relations are necessary whether the trades are unionized or not. Any strike, whether at the national or local level, will cause problems, with settlement on an individual project basis. If a project will involve the use of union labor, a general contingency plan should be developed to minimize the interruption and disruption of activities if a strike occurs.

Owners must also be observant in meeting their responsibilities. One is to provide sufficient and appropriate insurance for the project (e.g., for personal injuries; additional fire coverage). Insurance company representatives can be expected to inspect the project periodically. Another is making sure the contractor is bonded in the event that work cannot be completed. Bonding insures that a project will be completed under these circumstances. It is also applicable to subcontractors. An argument that not bonding will save the owner some money should be viewed with skepticism: it takes only one failure to ruin a project.

All of the preceding items involve paperwork and the signing of contracts. Owners and contractors should each maintain a file of all documents relating to the maintenance of safety. It will be useful to inspecting authorities; it will become critical in the event of an unfortunate incident.

NOTES

1. The difference between a minor and a major change cannot be specified. It is akin to trying to define a "small" hospital. Factors include the amount, the extent, and the need. Any proposed change must be addressed. The issue here is whether, and what, action is or can be taken.

CHAPTER 15

Final Approval, Licensure, and Start-up

Construction is now complete, and all inspections and reviews listed in Chapter 14 have been completed. Can the new structure now be occupied? Not quite. Several final approvals are necessary, and they are the subject of this chapter.

> **NOTE:** A complete file of all approvals should be kept by the owner. When an original copy of approval is required to be posted (e.g., an elevator permit), a duplicate copy should be kept on file.

WHO ISSUES FINAL APPROVALS?

There are two government agencies whose approval must be obtained in order to occupy and operate a new or renovated health care facility.

One is the state licensure agency, which issues a form, or license, stating what type or level of health care activity is permitted in the structure. This license is issued by the department of public health of the state (or sometimes county) after it makes a final inspection.

The other agency is the local building department in whose jurisdiction work was done. This department issues an occupancy permit, which, as the name implies, allows the owner to occupy and function in the structure.

If a facility will be treating patients whose bills will be paid through the Medicare and/or Medicaid program, then the approval of the Joint Commission on Accreditation of Healthcare Organizations (JCAHO) will be necessary.[1] Through JCAHO survey procedures, a facility can become accredited. The U.S. Department of Health and Human Services, which administers the Medicare and Medicaid programs, accepts JCAHO accreditation as a sign of meeting certain levels of operations and code compliance.

> **NOTE:** Although JCAHO is a nongovernment organization, the survey it conducts is not free. Owners must pay a fee. Further in connection with accreditation, a statement of construction from JCAHO must be completed and a field inspection made of the facility following construction.

WHO IS RESPONSIBLE FOR GETTING APPROVALS?

The owner is responsible for contacting the preceding agencies (and any others that are necessary) when the architect/engineer and contractor agree that work on the project has been completed. A mutually convenient date for all (owner, architect/engineer, contractor, and agencies) should be arranged for the final walk-through and inspections.

WHO WILL NEED TO SIGN THE APPROVALS?

The various agencies mentioned previously will need to sign their respective forms following approval. In some instances, an agency will require the owner (or his or her legally authorized representative) to sign as well. Some agencies require an affidavit from a testing company or licensed engineer affirming that a system, such as a fire alarm or sprinkler system, has been installed properly and tested and found to operate according to manufacturer specifications or local regulations.

ACTIVATING THE VARIOUS UTILITIES

As part of final approval, the hookup, activation, and checkout of the various utilities are necessary. These include electricity, gases, water, fire lines, steam, sewer, and drainage.

> **NOTE:** There are charges associated with making these connections, and the owner is responsible for paying them.

Electricity (Normal)

The contractor or subcontractor is responsible for adhering to local power company regulations. Final connections through the meter will be accomplished jointly between the contractor and the power company.

Electricity (Emergency)

An operational test must be conducted of the emergency system that is used if normal electric power is interrupted.[2] Health care facilities require some type of system to automatically restore electrical power to certain electrical equipment and receptacles.[3] The test must be conducted in the presence of the contractor, electrical engineer, local power company officials, the manufacturer (or a representative) of any prime mover and generator that is used, and the owner. This test is conducted to ensure both that the electric power so generated does not interfere with the electric power delivered by the utility company and that the system works when it is needed during an emergency. The test is conducted *after* normal electric power has been activated.

> **NOTE:** A vital part of the contract covering electric power is training facility personnel in the use of the main switch gear used to transfer from normal to emergency power.

Gases

As with electricity, adherence to local gas company regulations is the responsibility of the contractor or subcontractor. In addition, all gas lines and equipment must be tested and approved prior to actual use and testing. The gas company will do the actual turning on of gas. For gas-fired boilers, it is mandatory that the gas company turn the gas on.

> **WARNING:** For dual oil and gas systems, boilers must be purged prior to being turned on.

Water

Local water (public works) authorities, in cooperation with the contractor or subcontractor, make the final connection for water and sewer lines. In some instances, the city or town will make all the final connections, as well as do the work beyond the property lines (there will be a charge for this work). Where wells or private systems are used (i.e., where there are no public water lines), it is necessary for the contractor to do all the work, though under very strict regulations and inspection by local authorities.

Fire Lines

In a growing number of communities today, the water lines for fire suppression systems (i.e., for standpipes and sprinkler systems) are being installed separately from domestic (regular) water lines. Final connections for these lines are supervised by the department of public works, with the same procedures followed as for water lines. In some instances, the local fire department reviews the installation.

Steam

In some major cities (e.g., Boston), steam is supplied and regulated by the public works department and the power company. The final connection and testing of steam lines are conducted or supervised by the heating and ventilating contractor. The presence of local authorities may be required when this testing is conducted.

Sewer

Procedures for sewer connections are similar to those for water line connections. To be sure, sewer line connections must be completed *before* water lines are activated.

> **NOTE:** Some localities are proposing separate systems for sanitary sewer and storm sewer. In anticipation, localities may require new facilities to provide two lines to the street for future separate connection.

All Connections to Equipment

It is strongly recommended that qualified persons install and check plant equipment, such as vacuum pumps, air compressors, and chillers. Instruction on the use and maintenance of such equipment should be obtained. To aid in reviewing these instructions, or to orient future employees, a videotape of any presentations should be made and kept on file.

THE "PUNCH LIST"

In the final stages of construction, there will come a time when a very methodical walk-through of the project will be made with the owner, architect, engineers, and contractor. The purpose of this tour is to learn if everything in the contract is done or about to be done, or if anything is done incorrectly. The last two items generate what has come to be known as the punch list—a written agenda listing how, when, and at what cost (if any) these two items will be completed.

This probably sounds like a reasonable thing to do for any size project. Beware! Punch lists can be very aggravating, particularly when there are differences of opinion as to whether a particular item is indeed done or done incorrectly. If tempers rise high enough, the original coinage of the term may break out. It is hoped, of course, that discussions and differences would never degenerate to this level.

After the punch list is generated, a constant check of progress is made by the clerk of the works to be sure as many items as possible are completed when the owner takes formal possession of the area or structure. If any items are not completed at take-over time, they must be noted in writing as to how, when, and by whom they are to be completed.

With that, a project is technically, but not quite, completed. There are some activities and follow-up that need to be accomplished, which are detailed in the next chapter.

NOTES

1. Until 1988, JCAHO was JCAH, the Joint Commission on Accreditation of Hospitals. Originally, JCAH who formed to survey and accredit only hospitals. Over the years, other types of facilities were added. The list now includes hospices, pyschiatric facilities, long-term care facilities, ambulatory health care facilities, alcoholic and drug abuse facilities, and facilities serving the mentally retarded or developmentally handicapped. To reflect this expansion, JCAH changed its name to JCAHO.

2. The formal term for *emergency electric power* is *essential electricity*. The system for generating and distributing this electricity is termed the essential electrical system. Electricity itself is not an emergency quantity; it is the delivery of electric power from an alternate source, to

restore and continue *essential* services in an emergency when normal electric power has been interrupted, that is being accomplished.

3. The extent of restoration of electric power will depend on the type of medical care being provided. The most widely referenced document listing what is to be restored for different types of facilities is NFPA 99, Standard for Health Care Facilities. (In the 1984 edition of NFPA 99, see Chapter 8. In the 1987 edition of NFPA 99, see Chapters 12 through 18.)

CHAPTER 16

Postconstruction

Responsibilities for a health care facility project do not just end when construction is complete. There are important additional details to be handled following construction.

DEDICATION

As asked in Chapter 13, why hold a ceremony to formally announce to everyone that a facility is open? The answer is the same as before, but with an added factor: instead of marking what will be built, a dedication is honoring what has been built. It acknowledges the pride in accomplishing a goal — particularly one that is intended to serve the sick, aged, and/or handicapped in the community.

Because a dedication ceremony is similar to a ground-breaking ceremony, the same outline used in Chapter 13 is repeated in this section. Once again, if a dedication ceremony is held, it should be carried out well.

Why Bother?

As with a ground-breaking ceremony, there are no requirements or regulations that a dedication ceremony be held. It is a tradition dating back to antiquity. It is another formal marker in the building process, denoting that construction has been completed. It is also time to publicly call attention to those who helped make the project possible. Finally, it allows the public to see and become familiar with what has just been built.

Planning

Just about the same criteria prevail for planning a dedication ceremony as for planning a ground-breaking ceremony. Although a ground breaking usually starts before any serious construction commences, a dedication can take place near completion or even up to several months *after* the structure is occupied and activities have commenced. It is more common to delay a dedication so that staff have had an opportunity to get used to the new structure or area and create a smoothly running operation. Also, considering weather and the time of the year, an early spring dedication is preferable to a late winter one in many parts of the country.

Invitees

The same sensitivity toward invitations applies to a dedication as to a ground-breaking ceremony (see Chapter 13).

The Media

If good rapport with the media was established at the time of ground breaking and periodic contact has been maintained, then media coverage should not be a problem at dedication time. As before, the media should be provided with as much advance notice of the event as possible and with as much information about the sequence of events for the day. Some media may even ask to come hours or even a day early in order to tour the facility and take pictures at a more casual pace and in a more natural atmosphere.

If any problems or incidents occurred at any time prior or if picketing is anticipated, the media most assuredly will be present. In this instance, cooperation with the media is critical in order to gain at least balanced coverage. Trying to fight or ignore the media will only make the situation worse. On the other hand, equal time should be requested to present the facility's point of view: the media have the obligation to report both sides' views of a problem, and they can be challenged if one of the parties believes impartiality has been breached.

Logistics for the Day

In addition to all that was stated under this section in Chapter 13, arrangements for tours or walk-throughs of the facility will have to be made.

Depending on the size and capabilities of the structure and on the anticipated size of the crowd, an indoor dedication ceremony is preferable to an outdoor one since weather conditions will not have to be contended with. It will also allow more control over sound and lighting conditions.

The Ceremony

Tradition has established that a ribbon be cut as a mark of officially dedicating a new facility. Other than that, anything goes — within reason. Dedications commonly include champagne, a cake (sometimes in the shape of the new structure), a small momento for attendees.

Creativity and originality will go a long way toward having attendees remember the day and making a good impression in their minds. Hence, good taste should be exercised. And any problems that arise should be handled maturely.

THE WARRANTY PERIOD

Health care facility construction is no different from anything else in terms of assurance that the structure and equipment purchased will function for a period of time without trouble or, if some problem does arise, will be corrected under terms listed in a warranty agreement. There will therefore be warranties on construction and equipment for the project. The responsibility to obtain them rests with the contractor.

No one warranty will cover everything associated with a project. There are too many different items involved: those associated with construction (e.g., structural considerations; finishing work) and those items purchased by the contractor (e.g., equipment). Warranties themselves will vary for a host of reasons, such as the type of material, type of wear, maintenance, care, time, and use. Quite a few warranties, then, result from a project.

Most equipment warranties extend from 90 days to 1 year following owner acceptance and taking possession of an area or the structure. On large or complex equipment, the warranty could extend for as much as 2 years. Some equipment warranties cover parts and labor; others cover only parts.

Most contractors will warrant their general construction for a year, though with some limitations. This is not to say that poor construction is exempt from recompense after a year. The courts have been adamant about poor work and its correction by contractors.

For items purchased directly by the owner, the warranty is strictly between the owner and the seller. The general contractor would be responsible only for any connections made at the time of installation.

Thus, it is very important that a warranty list be assembled by the contractor that specifies exactly what will be warranted, for

how long, and if there are any limitations. This list should be
included in the specification book and reviewed by the archi-
tect/engineer and the owner. A signed copy of each warranty
should be kept on file by all parties.

A warranty list should also be assembled by the owner for all
equipment not purchased by the contractor. A copy of these
warranties should also be kept on file.

PAYMENTS

Payment should be thoroughly discussed during contract negotiations so that it does not become an embarrassing subject later.
As such, a payment schedule should be included in any contract.

There is no set method of payment for services of architects,
engineers, and contractors; payments will depend on what is
mutually satisfactory between all parties.

Architect/Engineer Fees

Although design of a building is generally completed well before
construction, payment of architectural fees is generally spread
out over the entire design and construction period. This is due, in
part, to the involvement of the architect throughout the construction period and even afterward.

Of the many payment schedules, two of the more common
ones are as follows. Both are developed after the lump-sum or
percentage-basis fee is agreed upon.

The first method could be termed *marker points*. A certain
percentage (based on the architect/engineer fees, not the total
construction cost) is paid at the completion of preliminary
sketches (e.g., 20 percent); a certain percentage is paid at the
completion of basic scale (design development) drawings (e.g., 20
percent); a certain percentage is paid after completion of working
drawings (e.g., 40 percent); and the remainder is paid over the
time of construction (such as monthly or quarterly payments).
The actual breakdown of percentages must be agreed upon during contract discussions.

The second method could be termed the *equal monthly installments*, or cash flow, method. It is the total amount of architectural fees divided by the total number of months anticipated to
design and build (or renovate) a facility. Since this method is
based on a projected time for completion, the monthly amount
can be adjusted as construction progresses and a firmer comple-

tion date is realized. This method of payment can be better for both parties, since a known *cash flow* will be established (both outgoing for the owner and incoming for the architect/engineer).

Contractor Fees

As with architectural fees, contractor fees and schedules of payments must be discussed and agreed upon during contract negotiations. Likewise, there are various methods that are used in making payments, depending on the construction method used (see Chapter 14 for a discussion of various construction methods). The following are two of the more common methods used.

> **NOTE:** Subcontractors are generally paid by the prime contractor. In some government contracts, the subcontractors are paid directly.

In the construction manager method, two types of payments are used. The first is payment to the construction manager for financial management of the project. This usually involves a down payment of about 10 percent of the total fee, with the remainder spread out over the period of design and construction. The second type of payment to the construction manager is in terms of construction work performed. Payment here is accomplished by a requisition submitted as each part, or a portion, of the construction is completed. (In many cases, this is done monthly.) The requisition, which must be signed by the construction manager, the architect, and the owner, will describe the work done as well as any costs for material purchased by the construction manager.[1]

With a straight bid contract, payments are made to the contractor by submission of requisitions that, again, describe the work done by the contractor and/or subcontractors and the materials stored, paid for, or used. In addition to the contractor, the architect and owner must sign the requisition. In some instances, if loans are involved, the lending institution may require its signature on the requisition. (This is for control purposes.) With this method, payments are of varying amounts throughout the construction period.

Payment for Other Construction Methods

For other construction methods, payment schedules are still similar to those mentioned previously. These other methods include the design/build method, in which the architect and builder are the same firm or are in partnership with each other; and the owner/contractor method, in which the owner acts as his or her own contractor and pays subcontractors.

Final Payment
In most contracts, a 10 percent final payment is withheld from a contractor for 30 days after acceptance of the area or structure by the owner for the purpose of clearing any and all final problems.

DOCUMENTATION

Documenting the construction or renovation of a health care facility is another important aspect of the building process. It provides a record of exactly what was built and how it was accomplished. This is useful information to have available should problems or questions arise or should further expansion or renovations be desired at some later date. Otherwise, unnecessary and additional costs would probably have to be expended to learn about these details. The information also reinforces the adage that those who do not learn from history are condemned to repeat it.

Storing Data
Documentation means more than just a set of drawings of what was built. Rather it is a set of information describing a process in its entirety. As such, this information should be organized so as to make its retrieval relatively easy. Hence, a well-organized filing system should be established from the beginning of a project.

Today, stored information includes not only hard copy but also microfiches, computer disks and diskettes, and videotape cassettes. Because of the extensiveness of some projects, any or all of these storage mechanisms may be necessary just because of the lack of space in which to store the amount of hard copy that is generated.

What Should be Stored?
Documentation can consist of any or all of the following, depending on the extensiveness of the project. (It is not in chronological or priority order.) All should be in a form, however, that makes reproduction relatively easy.

1. Construction photographs. These are required to document progress and should be made during construction. Problems, in particular, should be photographed for future reference. Before and after photographs should be included.

2. Copy of any long- and short-range studies or planning that was conducted in connection with the project. It is very easy to forget after a few years where the project fit into the grand scheme of things and why certain planning was done. The original persons involved may not be available to answer questions.

3. Copy of any feasibility studies.

4. Copy of the Certificate of Need (CON) procedures that were followed and those CONs that were approved.

5. Set of all contracts (architectural, contractor, subcontractor, requisitions, and purchase orders.[2]

6. Full set of updated as-built drawings reflecting actual construction (see Chapter 12). Associated with this package is the specification book, all change orders, and detailed drawings.

7. Copy of the daily log kept by the clerk of the works.

8. Record of all payments to the architect, contractor, and subcontractor. This includes payments to the clerk of the works.

9. Record of external costs. These are purchases made by the owner directly for equipment and material for the project.

10. Set of all approvals from all agencies, organizations, and companies that were necessary or were involved in the project.

11. Set of all warranty agreements.

12. Copy or set of instructions for all equipment. This can include videotapes, brochures, and user and maintenance manuals.

13. File of all legal and other financial costs (e.g., lawyer fees, surveyor fees, court costs).

14. List of addresses and telephone numbers of all pertinent

agencies, persons, companies, and other groups involved in the project.

15. Organized file of all correspondence, meetings (including minutes when appropriate), and notes associated with the project.

This documentation may seem burdensome and too paper oriented. However a well-organized file and filing system will save immeasurable time (and thus money) in later years when trying to locate information for internal needs as well for external requests or audits.

NOTES

1. The signing of the requisition by all three major parties (architect/ engineer, contractor, and owner) is necessary to preclude later legal problems regarding lack of knowledge of the requisition.

2. Requisitions and purchase orders are forms of contracts.

Appendix A
Code Review Procedures Checklist
(New Construction Only)

The following checklist has been developed so that readers can see in outline form just how many agencies have jurisdiction over health care facilities and can require plans and other documents before work can commence on a project. Readers are cautioned that this list may not be complete for their particular project or locality.

Some points to consider:

1. Be sure project is health care related before using this checklist.

2. If project is health care related, determine the type of occupancy (e.g., hospital, nursing home, supervisory care facility).

3. Special health care facilities (e.g., physical rehabilitation, drug abuse, clinic) warrant caution as to the exact levels of codes and regulations to use.

4. Each project is unique. Do not assume a particular project is like any other.

I. CERTIFICATE OF NEED (CON)
   A. Project over $_____ (varies for each state) _____ [ ]
   B. Change of service _____ [ ]
   C. New service _____ [ ]
   D. Contact _____ [ ]
   E. Plan approval _____ [ ]
   F. Financial forms that must be submitted _____ [ ]

II. ARCHITECT/DESIGNER CODE REVIEW
   A. Initial early-on concept review _____ [ ]
   B. Preliminary-sketch-level review _____ [ ]
   C. Basic-scale-level review (design development)____ [ ]
   D. Working-drawing-level review (bidding) _____ [ ]
   E. Specifications review _____ [ ]

III. AGENCY REVIEWS
  A. Local (e.g., city, town)

> **NOTE:** 1. Time frame for review is from design development drawings through working-level drawings. 2. Signed approval should be obtained from all pertinent authorities. 3. Review should be done at least twice: at the beginning and at the end. For larger, more complicated projects, it is advised that a review be obtained at the preliminary schematic level and include proposed site work.

  1. Zoning ————————————————— [ ]
  2. Traffic control ————————————— [ ]
  3. Public works (e.g., sewer, water drainage, gas, electric, curb cuts) ——————————————— [ ]
  4. Environmental (e.g., wetlands, pollution control, local problems) ——————————————— [ ]
  5. Building department ————————— [ ]
  6. Fire department (e.g., fire zone determination) —— [ ]
  B. State and/or County

> **NOTE:** 1. Building codes and editions used vary from state to state. 2. Handicapped codes vary from state to state. 3. Most states have adopted U.S. Department of Health and Human Services regulations to some degree and use them as gudes in reviews or as actual legisled code. The edition used, however, varies from state to state. 4. NFPA 101, Life Safety Code, is used in every state, either as is or as an edited Fire Code (a document used for protecting people from fire and associated hazards). The edition used, however, varies from state to state.

  1. Department of public safety ——————— [ ]
  2. Department of public health (sometimes the department of labor and industry. ——————— [ ]

> **NOTE:** The following list is not all-inclusive and may vary from state to state.

    a. Radiological control and licensure ————— [ ]

b. Intensive care unit/cardiac care unit —————— [ ]
c. Newborn licensure ————————————— [ ]
d. Long-term care licensure ————————— [ ]
e. Rehabilitation licensure ————————— [ ]
f. Handicapped regulations (may be in building department) ———————————————— [ ]
g. Mental health licensure and approval ———— [ ]
h. Alcohol drug rehabilitation approval ———— [ ]
3. CON review ————————————————— [ ]

NOTE: 1. This may be the department of public health in some states. 2. This requires submission of plans and specifications that first must be approved by local building departments and state departments of public safety.

4. State environmental (e.g., wetlands, sewer, drainage, air pollution, water pollution) ———————— [ ]
5. State parks ———————————————— [ ]
6. State highways ——————————————— [ ]
7. State rights of way ————————————— [ ]
8. The state agency for the following should be determined and information forwarded to the responsible engineer.
   a. Boiler inspection, review, approval ———— [ ]
   b. Fuel tank review and approval ————— [ ]
   c. Medical gas review and approval ———— [ ]
   d. Asbestos removal (existing structures only; not used in new construction)
   e. Energy review and approval: energy audit —— [ ]
                                lighting audit —— [ ]
   f. Subsoil and concrete testing ——————— [ ]
   g. Earthquake control ———————————— [ ]
   h. Gas fuel inspection approval ——————— [ ]
C. Federal Agencies
   1. Joint Commission on Accreditation of Healthcare Organizations (JCAHO) —————————————— [ ]

NOTE: 1. JCAHO is not a federal agency. However, the U.S. Department of Health and Human Services accepts JCAHO accreditation. 2. JCAHO now surveys more than hospital-related facilities.
   2. Navigational (aircraft) control ——————— [ ]

NOTE: 1. Depends on location of structure. 2. Formerly under Federal Aviation Administration (FAA); now under Department of Transportation.

3. CON—Federal level ———————————————— [ ]

NOTE: Requirements are set for the local level. Federal approval is generally pro forma.

IV. STATE-OWNED PROJECTS

NOTE: 1. State can set its own criteria. 2. Specific criteria codes must be determined. 3. Adjacent federal lands may have an impact at the start of the project.

A. Name of agency ———————————————— [ ]
B. Codes and regulations used ————————————

———————————————————————————

———————————————————————————

V. FEDERAL PROJECTS

NOTE: 1. Each agency or department (e.g., Veterans' Administration, Army, Air Force, Navy, Public Health) can set its own criteria. 2. Specific criteria and codes must be determined. 3. Adjacent federal lands may have an impact at the start of the project.

A. Name of agency/dept. ———————————— [ ]
B. Codes and regulations used ———————————— [ ]

Appendix B
General Evaluation and Checklist
For Any Existing Building

This checklist is applicable to any building, either a health care facility or a building being converted to a health care facility. (See Appendix C for an additional checklist for a health care facility.)

Basic Structure Type _____

Materials:
    Concrete _____ Steel (fireproofed) _____ Wood _____
    Exterior Finish _____
    Roof Construction _____
    Window Type(s) _____
    Window Size(s) _____
    Special Features _____
_____

Basic Size and Shape _____
    Height _____
    No. of stories: Above grade _____ Below grade _____

Zoning
    Front yard setback _____
    Rear yard setback _____
    Left side yard setback _____
    Right side yard setback _____

Utilities
    Water, domestic _____
    Water, fire _____ Building connection _____
    Sewer, sanitary _____
    Sewer, drainage _____
    Electric _____
    Gas _____
    Telephone _____
    Television _____
    Alarms _____

Parking Facilities
   Normal (patients, staff, visitors) _____
   Handicapped _____
   Emergency _____
   Lighting _____
   Access _____

Description of Terrain (trees, shrubs, grade) _____
_____
_____
_____

Building Interior (each floor and its use) _____
_____
_____

Interior Egress (describe how)
   Corridor _____
   Exit doors _____
   Ramps _____
   Stairs _____

Rating or Fire-Resistance Level of Exits _____
_____
_____

Handicapped: Conditions of Exit and Access _____
_____
_____

Fire Alarms
   Audible _____ Visual _____
Smoke Alarms _____
Heat Detectors _____
   Tied to fire alarm system? _____
Sprinklers _____ Standpipes _____
Pull Stations _____
   Within 5 feet of exits? _____
Roof Access (for fire department) _____
Fire Fighting Equipment _____
_____

Interior Partitions (describe for each area)
Corridors _____
Rooms _____
Public facilities _____
Stairs _____
Shafts _____

NOTE: Include floor, walls, base, dado, and ceilings.

Heating, Ventilating, and Air Conditioning System(s) (describe, indicating existence of fire and smoke dampers) _____
_____
_____
_____

Plumbing (describe, including gas) _____
_____
_____

Electric (describe) _____
_____
_____
_____

Emergency Generator(s) (describe, including size and capacity)
_____
_____

Emergency Lighting (describe)
On generator(s) _____
_____
On battery(ies) _____
_____

Low-voltage System(s): Intercom, Music, Paging, Closed-Circuit Television, Radio (describe) _____
_____
_____

Basic Service Company (name, telephone number, contact) ____
_____

Goods Receiving Area
Doors — height _____
Door size _____
Turnaround for large trucks _____
Parking for salespeople _____
Separate road access and exit _____
_____

Fuel receiving _____
Trash removal _____
Laundry _____
Food _____
Medical goods _____
Gas (propane, oxygen, etc.) _____
_____

General goods _____
Storage space _____
Offices _____
Uncrating and sorting _____

Workshops
Carpentry _____
HVAC _____
Plumbing _____
Electric _____

Engineering
Offices (include toilets, showers, and lockers) _____
_____

Mechanical spaces _____

General Condition of Existing Building(s): (describe, indicating
any deterioration, such as leaky roof, cracked concrete, trim rot,
extreme interior wear (particularly floors, doors, walls), or reme-
dial work needed, such as on brick pointing, windows, door
weather stripping) _____
_____
_____
_____
_____
_____

Appendix C
Evaluation and Checklist
For Existing Health Care Facilities

The following is a general checklist for health care facilities. It may not indicate all items or cover any particular institution. It is intended to assist a designer or surveyor in reviewing an existing institution. Checking off the items noted provides a better understanding of existing features.

> **NOTE:** All items listed in the general survey for existing buildings (Appendix B), such as sprinklers, smoke detectors, pull stations, alarms, room finishes, fire ratings, lighting levels, heating, ventilating, emergency electrical power, and miscellaneous plumbing features, are not repeated in this appendix. The following information, therefore, should be determined for the specific health care facility, in addition to the general items covered in Appendix B.

I. ADMINISTRATIVE AREAS
  A. Lobby/waiting area. Will require the following:
    1. Receptionist _____ Directory _____
    2. Public toilets: Male ____ Female ____ Handicapped ____
    3. Public telephones _____ Handicapped _____
    4. Drinking fountains _____ Handicapped _____
    5. Wheelchair waiting space _____
  B. Offices and administrative spaces
    1. Administrative offices _____
    2. Interview
      a. Patient _____
      b. Employee _____
    3. Business office(s)
      a. Cashier _____
      b. Accounting _____
      c. Data processing _____
    4. Records (files)
      a. Medical _____

    b. Business _____
    5. Library
        a. Medical _____
        b. Other _____
    6. Chiefs of services (medical/surgical offices) _____
    7. Mail room _____
    8. Purchasing _____
    9. Receiving _____
    10. Central stores _____
    11. Engineering (facility/clinical) _____
    12. Trades ("shops") _____
    13. Employees
        a. Toilets _____ b. Showers _____
        c. Lockers _____ d. Restrooms _____
    14. Grounds maintenance _____
    15. Housekeeping
        a. Janitor closets _____
        b. Floor storage _____
        c. Cart sanitizing _____
    16. Work flow pattern for all departments _____
    _____

II. CENTRAL SUPPLY (MEDICAL AND SURGICAL)
    A. Receiving and cleanup _____
    B. Clean work area _____
    C. Storage _____
        1. Clean _____ 2. Unsterile _____
        3. Cart _____
    D. Sewing space _____
    E. Sterilizer types:
        1. Steam _____ 2. Gas (vented) _____

III. DETOXIFICATION UNITS
    A. Bedroom size _____
    B. Patient toilets _____
        1. Emergency pull-cord (nurse use only) _____
    C. Corridor size _____
    D. Education rooms _____
    E. Recreation rooms _____
    F. Adjunct facilities (if shared):
        1. Radiology _____
        2. Laboratory (urinalysis/hematology) _____

IV. DIETARY
  A. Kitchen
    1. Cooking area:
      a. Hoods ——————————————————————
      b. Fire control ————————————————————
    2. Washable ceilings/walls ————————————————
    3. Nonslip floors ————————————————————
    4. Location of fire extinguishers ——————————————
  B. Employees
    1. Toilets (not in kitchen) ——————————————————
    2. Hand washing (in kitchen) ————————————————
      a. No mirror ——————————————————————
    3. Lockers ——————————————————————
    4. Restrooms ——————————————————————
  C. Serving area ——————————————————————
  D. Dining area ——————————————————————
  E. Storage
    1. Refrigerators ——————————————————————
    2. Daily stores ——————————————————————
    3. Bulk storage ——————————————————————
  F. Coffee shop ——————————————————————
  G. Vending ——————————————————————
  H. Floor nourishment (patient) ————————————————
  I. Floor kitchen (patient) ——————————————————
  J. Janitor closets required for kitchen use only ——————————
    ——————————————————————
  K. Dish washing (water temperature) ———————————————
  L. Waste method ——————————————————————
  M. Ice (dietary) ——————————————————————

V. EMERGENCY
  A. Control ——————————————————————
    1. Outpatient Department ———————— 2. Emergency ————————
  B. Waiting space
    1. Drinking fountains (handicapped) ——————————————
    2. Public toilets (handicapped) ————————————————
    3. Public telephones ——————————————————————
  C. Interview space ——————————————————————
  D. Wheelchair/litter space ————————————————————
  E. Triage area
    1. Scrub-up ———————— 2. Equipment ————————

F. Cast room
  1. Plaster trap/sink _____
  2. X-ray view _____
  3. Gases _____
G. First-aid spaces
  1. Hand washing _____ 2. Gases _____
  3. Storage spaces _____
  4. Nurse emergency call _____
H. Trauma
  1. Hand washing _____ 2. Gases _____
  3. Electric _____ 4. Intravenous track _____
 I. Minor operating room
  1. Scrub-up _____ 2. Gases _____
  3. Electric _____ 4. X-ray view _____
  5. Intravenous track _____
J. Observation room(s)
  1. Check need _____
K. Staff toilets _____
L. Business
  1. Admissions _____
  2. Files/records _____
M. Drug control _____
N. Soiled work room _____
  1. Hand washing _____
O. Clean work room _____
  1. Hand washing _____
P. Dressing booths (patients) _____
  1. Size _____
Q. Corridors _____
  1. Width _____ 2. Ceiling height _____

VI. INTENSIVE CARE UNIT (ICU)/CARDIAC CARE UNIT
(CCU)
  A. Patient (bed) area (ICU)
    1. Size _____ 2. Gases _____
    3. Nurse emergency call ____ 4. Intravenous track____
    5. Clock _____ Calendar _____
    7. Window _____ Borrowed light _____
    9. Toilet facility _____
    10. Hand washing _____
    11. Monitors _____

B. Patient (bed) area (CCU)
   1. Size _____ Gases _____
   3. Nurse emergency call _____ 4. Intravenous track _____
   5. Clock _____ 6. Calendar _____
   7. Toilet facility _____
   8. Hand washing _____
   9. Monitors _____
C. Nurses' station _____
   1. View of patient _____
   2. Charting _____
   3. Monitors _____
   4. Hand washing _____
   5. Adjacent toilet _____ Restroom _____
D. Drug station _____
E. Clean utility room _____
   1. Hand washing _____
   2. Counter _____ 3. Sink _____
F. Soiled utility
   1. Hand washing _____
   2. Bedpan facility _____
   3. Flushing room sink _____
G. Nourishment station _____
   1. Hand washing _____
   2. Ice _____ 3. Refrigeration _____
H. Patient clothing storage _____
 I. Waiting area (visitors) _____
   1. Public telephones _____
 J. Staff lockers _____
K. Corridors _____
   1. Width _____ 2. Height _____

VII. LABORATORIES (See also Bibliography, in particular "Code Manual for Health Care Facility," published by The Ritchie Organization)
   A. Type
      1. Chemistry _____
      2. Bacteriology _____
      3. Miscellaneous _____
   B. Checks in general
      1. Hoods (venting) _____
      2. Gas storage (cylinders) _____

    3. Piped gas systems _____
    4. Air supply and exhaust _____
    5. Refrigeration _____
    6. Electrical loading _____
    7. Eye washers _____ 8. Emergency showers _____
    9. Fire blankets _____
  C. Blood bank _____
    1. Refrigeration _____
    2. Hand washing _____
    3. Donor room _____
  D. Dedicated janitor closets _____
  E. Cleanup room _____

VIII. MORGUE
  A. Body room/refrigerators _____
  B. Autopsy room _____
    1. Hood (venting) _____
    2. Hand washing _____
    3. Flushing-rim service sink _____
    4. Table and drain _____

IX. LAUNDRY
  A. Soiled area _____
    1. Hand washing _____
  B. Clean area _____
  C. Dedicated janitor closets _____
  D. Size of laundry _____
    1. Over 1,000 square feet, 2 exits _____
  E. Receiving (if not in house) _____
  F. Laundry chutes _____
    1. Class of construction/B label fire doors _____

X. NEWBORN
  A. Nursery type _____
    1. Full-term _____
    2. Isolation _____
    3. Special care _____
    4. Premature _____
  B. Checks in general _____
    1. Size of room _____ 2. Capacity _____
    3. Hand washing _____
    4. Work space _____

    5. Gases (including compressed air) —————————
    6. Electric ————————————————————
    7. Work space/room ———————————————
      a. Hand washing ————— b. Refrigerator ————
    8. Dedicated janitor closets ————————————
    9. Treatment space ——————————————
   10. Baby viewing area ——————————————
 C. Parents' waiting area ——————————————
    1. Public telephone ——————————————
 D. Birthing rooms (see section XV, below)

XI. NURSING (LONG-TERM)
 A. Bedroom (patient) ———————————————
    1. Size ————— 2. Window (stool height) ————
    3. Toilet facility —————————————————
    4. Grab bars in toilet ———————————————
    5. Nurse emergency call in toilet ————————
 B. Treatment room ————————————————
    1. Size ————— 2. Hand washing ——————
    3. Desk ————————————————————
 C. Clean utility ——————————————————
    1. Hand washing ————————————————
    2. Counter sink —————————————————
 D. Soiled utility ——————————————————
    1. Hand washing ————————————————
    2. Flushing-rim service sink ————————————
 E. Janitor Closet(s) ————————————————
 F. Dayroom/recreation ———————————————
    1. Size ——————————————————————
 G. Dining space ——————————————————
    1. Size ————————————————————
    2. Hand washing ————————————————
    3. Drinking fountains (handicapped) ————————
 H. Nurses' station ————————————————
    1. Hand washing ————————————————
    2. Adjacent toilet ————————————————
    3. Clock —————————————————————
 I. Doctors' charting ————————————————
 J. Drug station ——————————————————
    1. Locking ————————————————————
 K. Staff ——————————————————————
    1. Toilets —————————————————————

2. Lockers ——————————————————————
3. Rest ——————————————————————————
L. Nurses' office ——————————————————————
M. Patient bathing ——————————————————————
  1. Showers ————————————————————————
  2. Baths ——————————————————————————
  3. Sitz ———————————————————————————
N. Linen (clean) ————————————————————————
O. Linen (soiled) ———————————————————————
P. Nourishment station ————————————————————
  1. Hand washing ————————————————————————
  2. Ice —————————— 3. Refrigeration ——————————
Q. Items such as personal care, physical therapy, and occupational therapy facilities can be shared.
R. Corridors ——————————————————————————
  1. Width —————————— 2. Height ————————————
S. Training toilet —————————————————————————
  1. Size —————————— 2. Clearance (3 feet) ——————
  3. Toilet —————————— 4. Shower ——————————————
  5. Bath —————————— 6. Grab bars ————————————
  7. Mirror ———————————————————————————

XII. NURSING (MEDICAL AND SURGICAL)

A. Room (patient bed)
  1. Size —————————— 2. Toilet facility ——————————
  3. Gases —————————— 4. Electric ————————————
  5. Nurse call ——— 6. Nurse emergency call (toilet) ———
  7. Window ————————— 8. Curtain track (bed) —————
  9. Intravenous track (bed) — 10. Window (stool height) —
B. Nurses' station
  1. Hand washing ————————— 2. Clock ——————————
  3. Adjacent toilet ——————————————————————
C. Doctors' charting ——————————————————————
D. Clean utility ————————————————————————
  1. Hand washing ————————————————————————
E. Soiled utility ————————————————————————
  1. Hand washing ——— 2. Flushing-rim service sink ———
F. Treatment room(s) ——————————————————————
  1. Hand washing —————————— 2. Desk ——————————
G. Patient bathing ————————————————————————
  1. Showers —————————— 2. Baths ——————————————
  3. Sitz ———————————————————————————

    H. Staff ——————————————————————
       1. Toilets ——————————————————————
       2. Rest ————————————— 3. Lockers ————————————
    I. Janitor closet(s) ——————————————————————
    J. Multipurpose room(s) ——————————————————————
    K. Isolation room ——————————————————————
       1. Size ——————————————————————
       2. Toilet ——————————————————————
       3. Bath ——————————————————————
    L. Detention room ——————————————————
       1. (Can be located in another area) ——————————————
       2. Size ————————————— 3. Toilet ————————————
    M. Nurses' office ——————————————————————
    N. Toilet (wheelchair) ——————————————————
       1. Grab bars ————————— 2. Emergency call————————
    O. Stretcher and wheelchair storage ——————————————
    P. Public telephone(s) (handicapped) ——————————————
    Q. Waiting area (visitors) ——————————————————
       1. Size ——————————————————————

XIII. NURSING (PSYCHIATRIC/SUPERVISORY CARE)
All items similar to Nursing (Medical and Surgical) with the
following exceptions:
    1. No nurse emergency call required ——————————————
    2. Consultation rooms provided ——————————————
    3. Size of dining, occupational therapy ——————————————
    4. Open area to corridors ——————————————————
    5. Type of glass in windows ——————————————————
    6. Locks ——————————————————————

XIV. OBSTETRICS
    A. Delivery room
       1. Size ————————————— 2. Gases ————————————
       3. Electric ————————————— 4. Lights ————————————
       5. X-ray view ————————— 6. Record board —————————
       7. Baby utilities station ——————————————————
       8. Adjacent scrub-up area ——————————————————
    B. Labor room ——————————————————————
       1. Size ————————————— 2. Hand washing ——————————
       3. Gases ————————— 4. Intravenous track —————————
       5. Bed curtains ————————— 6. Emergency call —————————
       7. Nurses' station visible ——————————————————

8. Toilet facilities _____ 9. Showers _____
10. Clock _____
C. Dedicated janitor closet _____
D. Nurses' control station
   1. Hand washing _____ 2. Adjacent toilet _____
   3. Clock _____ 4. Drug control unit _____
E. Recovery room
   1. Size _____ 2. Bed clearance _____
   3. Gases _____ 4. Electric _____
   5. Emergency call _____ 6. Supervision _____
F. Substerile _____
   1. Type of sterilizers _____
G. Soiled work room _____
   1. Hand washing _____ 2. Flushing-rim service sink _____
H. Clean work room _____
   1. Hand washing _____ 2. Counter/sink _____
I. Gas storage _____
   1. Piped _____ 2. Loose _____
                                      Flammable _____
                                       Nonflammable _____
J. Supervisor's office _____
K. Anesthesiologist's office _____
   1. Work room _____ 2. Gases _____
L. Storage _____
   1. Equipment _____ 2. Litters _____
M. Staff _____
   1. Lockers _____ 2. Toilets _____
     a. Male _____ b. Female _____
   3. Showers _____ 4. On-call room(s) _____
   5. Rest _____ 6. Nourishment _____

XV. BIRTHING ROOM
  A. Bedroom (patient)
     1. Size _____ 2. Window _____
     3. Clock _____ 4. Toilet facility _____
     5. Bathing facility _____ 6. Gases _____
     7. Electric _____ 8. Nurses call _____
     9. Emergency call (toilet) _____
     10. Emergency call (nurse only) _____
     11. Baby gas and electric station _____

XVI. OCCUPATIONAL/PHYSICAL THERAPY
A. Exercise/treatment area _____
  1. Hand washing (handicapped) _____
  2. Drinking fountain (handicapped) _____
  3. Curtains (privacy) _____
B. Dressing (patient) _____
  1. Dressing booths _____ 2. Toilets _____
  3. Showers _____
C. Janitor closet _____
D. Stretcher and wheelchair storage _____
E. Storage _____
  1. Equipment _____ 2. Paint _____
F. Soiled area _____
  1. Flushing-rim service sink _____
  2. Hand washing _____
G. Pool _____
  1. Water filtration system _____
H. Respiratory therapy _____
  1. Gases _____ 2. Hand washing _____
I. Corridors _____
  1. Width _____ 2. Height _____
J. Office(s) _____

XVII. OPERATING SUITE
A. Major operating room
  1. Size _____ 2. Gases _____
  3. Electric _____ 4. Lights _____
  5. Flooring _____ 6. Ceiling _____
  7. X-ray view _____ 8. Adjacent scrub _____
  9. Clock timer _____ 10. Clock _____
B. Minor operating room (Items are the same as for major operating room)
C. Cystoscopy and endoscopy _____
  1. X-ray unit with control _____
  2. Floor drain _____
  3. Remote control drain _____

(Remaining items are the same as for major operating room.)

D. Cast room _____
  1. Sink-trap for plaster _____ 2. Splint storage _____

(Remaining items are the same as for major operating room.)

E. Holding area (anesthesia preparation) _____
   1. Gases _____ 2. Electric _____
   3. Emergency call _____ 4. Privacy curtains _____
F. Recovery room _____
   1. Litter clearance _____ 2. Gases _____
   3. Electric _____ 4. Monitors _____
   5. Privacy curtains _____ 6. Supervision _____
   7. Drug control station _____ 8. Hand washing _____
   9. Flushing-rim service sink _____ (bedpan use)
G. Staff
   1. Toilets _____ 2. Showers _____
   3. Rest _____ 4. Nourishment _____
   5. On-call _____
H. Frozen section laboratory: special equipment _____
I. Janitor closet, dedicated _____
J. Clean work room _____
   1. Hand washing _____
K. Anesthesiologist _____ 1. Office _____
   2. Work room _____ 3. Gases _____
L. Supervisor's office _____
M. Nurses' control (area) _____
   1. Drug control _____
N. Stretcher control _____
O. Corridors: 1. Width _____ 2. Height _____
P. Storage _____
   1. Equipment _____ 2. Clean goods _____
Q. X-O-Mat space _____
   1. Venting _____
R. Substerile _____
   1. Sterilizers _____ 2. Blanket warmer _____
   3. Still _____ 3. Sinks _____
S. Day surgery
   1. Waiting area _____

(Remaining items are similar to items for major operating room.)

XVIII. OUTPATIENT AMBULATORY CARE
  A. Control station _____
  B. Waiting area _____
   1. Clock _____ 2. Size _____
   3. Public telephone (handicapped) _____

    4. Drinking fountain (handicapped) _____

5. Toilets (handicapped) _____ 6. Wheelchair space _____

    C. Litter/wheelchair storage _____

    D. Treatment spaces/rooms _____

       1. Size _____ 2. Hand washing _____

       3. X-ray view _____ 4. Privacy _____

    E. Clean utility _____

       1. Hand washing _____ 2. Counter sink _____

    f. Soiled utility _____

       1. Hand washing _____ 2. Flushing-rim service sink _____

    G. Interview

       1. Privacy _____ 2. Credit _____

       3. Social service _____ 4. Business _____

       5. Medical records _____

    H. Emergency equipment _____

       1. Space size _____ 2. Utilities _____

    I. Police space _____

       1. Telephone _____

    J. Adjacency to laboratories, Radiology, other areas _____

XIX. PEDIATRICS

    A. Bedroom (patient) _____

       1. Size _____ 2. Gases _____

       3. Electric _____ 4. Privacy curtains _____

       5. View windows _____ 6. Windows _____

       7. Nurses' call (bed) ___ 8. Emergency call (nurse only) ___

       9. Toilet facilities _____

    B. Isolation (bedroom) _____

       1. Size _____ 2. Bath and toilet _____

       3. Anteroom _____

(Remaining items are the same as for regular bedrooms.)

    C. Nursery _____

       1. Size _____ 2. Gases _____

       3. Electric _____ 4. Anteroom _____

       5. Hand washing _____

    D. Treatment room _____

       1. Size _____ 2. Gases _____

       3. Desk _____ 4. X-ray view _____

    E. Dining space _____

       1. Hand washing _____

    F. Educational _____

G. Patient bathing _____
   1. Shower _____ 2. Bath _____
H. Storage _____
   1. Recreational items _____ 2. General _____
I. Formula preparation (see Nursery) _____
J. Wheelchair toilet _____
   1. Grab bars _____ 2. Emergency call (nurse only) _____
K. Corridors _____
   1. Width _____ 2. Height _____
L. Playroom _____

(See Educational, above.)

M. Family waiting _____
   1. Public telephone (handicapped) _____

XX. PHARMACY
A. Assembly area _____
   1. Hand washing _____ 2. Still _____
   3. Equipment _____ 4. Sinks _____
B. Office _____
C. Dispensing _____
D. Refrigerators _____
   1. Alarms _____
E. Drug room _____
   1. Size _____ 2. Alarms _____
F. Alcohol room _____
   1. Drain/storage _____
G. Storage (bulk) _____
   1. Security _____ 2. Intravenous storage _____
H. Laminar flow _____
I. Equipment _____
J. Janitor closet _____
K. Conference room _____
L. Staff _____
   1. Toilets _____ 2. Rest _____
   3. Nourishment _____ 4. Lockers _____
M. Corridors _____
   1. Width _____ 2. Height _____

XXI. RADIOLOGY AND IMAGING
A. Type of room
   1. Fluoroscopy _____ 2. Radiographic _____

3. Special procedures _____ 4. Cobalt _____
5. Magnetic resonance imaging _____ 6. CAT scanner _____
7. Linear scanner _____ 8. Ultrasound _____
9. Other _____ 10. As yet unknown _____
B. The following items should be checked for applicability to above areas

NOTE: Applies to treatment room *and* staff control room.

1. Lead _____
2. Electrical interference _____
3. Mass masonry _____
4. Earth _____
5. Magnetic _____
C. Toilet (fluoroscopic) _____
    1. Protection _____ 2. Grab bars _____
    3. Emergency call _____
D. Dressing (patient)
    1. Privacy _____ 2. Grab bars _____
    3. Emergency call _____
E. Waiting area
    1. Size _____ 2. Public telephone (handicapped) _____
    3. Drinking fountain (handicapped) _____
F. Control/information station _____
G. Holding area
    1. Space for litters _____ 2. Gases _____
    3. Electric _____ 4. Emergency call _____
    5. Privacy curtains _____
H. Offices _____
    1. X-ray view _____
I. Film processing _____
    1. Darkroom _____ 2. X-O-Mat space _____
J. Files and administration _____
    1. Storage units _____
K. Corridors
    1. Width _____ 2. Height _____

XXII. REHABILITATION
    A. Patient room
        1. Size _____ 2. Gases _____

3. Electric —————— 4. Window ——————
5. Toilet facilities ———— 6. Toilet grab bars ————
7. Nurse emergency call (toilet) ——————————
8. Emergency call (nurse only) ——————————
9. Nurses' call (bed)
B. Patient toilet/shower/bath ——————————
  1. Adjacent to room ——————————
  2. Training toilet ——————————
    a. Clearance ——————————
    b. Type of fixtures ——————————
    c. Grab bars ——————————
    d. Emergency call——————————
C. Special baths ——————————
  1. Type of unit ———— 2. Hand washing ————
  3. Emergency call———— 4. Grab bars ————
D. Nurses' station ——————————
  1. Clock ———— 2. Hand washing ————
  3. Adjacent toilet ——————————
E. Doctors' charting ——————————
F. Examination/treatment room ——————————
  1. Hand washing ———— 2. X-ray view ————
  3. Desk ——————————
G. Nurses' office ——————————
H. Storage ——————————
  1. Litters ———— 2. Wheelchairs ————
  3. Linen (clean) ———— 4. Linen (soiled) ————
  5. General equipment ——————————
I. Multipurpose room ——————————
  1. Size ——————————
J. Clean workroom ——————————
  1. Hand washing ———— 2. Counter sink ————
K. Soiled workroom ——————————
L. Nourishment ——————————
  1. Hand washing ———— 2. Ice ————
  3. Refrigeration ——————————
M. Janitor closet ——————————
N. Physical therapy and occupational therapy ————
  1. Hand washing (handicapped) ——————————
  2. Drinking fountain (handicapped) ——————————
  3. Privacy curtains ——————————
O. Hydrotherapy ——————————
  1. Pool ———— 2. Baths ————

    3. Other _____

  P. Dressing and showers (patient) _____

    1. Privacy _____ 2. Grab bars _____

    3. Emergency call _____

  Q. Corridors _____

    1. Width _____ 2. Height _____

  R. Speech and hearing _____

    1. Soundproofing _____ 2. Space size _____

  S. Prosthetics and orthotics _____

    1. Space size _____

  T. Dental unit _____

    1. Size _____ 2. Gases _____

    3. Electric _____ 4. Hand washing _____

  U. Dining and recreational (patient) _____

    1. Size _____ 2. Personal care _____

    3. Daily living activities (teaching) _____

    4. Psychological offices _____

    5. Social service offices _____

    6. Electrophoresis room _____

    7. Laboratory (can be in adjacent hospital) _____

  V. Vocational services unit _____

    1. Size _____ 2. Work space type _____

  W. Radiology unit (can be in adjacent hospital) _____

    1. Size _____ 2. Equipment _____

NOTE: If radiology unit is provided, see Section XXI, Radiology and Imaging

XXIII. WASTE PROCESSING

  A. Type of unit _____

    1. Incinerator _____

    2. Compactor _____

    3. Trash chute _____

    4. Destructor _____

    5. Can and bottle crusher _____

    6. Disposal(s) _____

  B. Rooms where units above are used _____

    1. Hose bib _____ 2. Venting _____

XXIV. VOLUNTEERS

  A. Offices _____ B. Lockers _____

  C. Toilets _____ D. Work space _____

Appendix D
Health Care Firesafety Compendium, 1987
Burton R. Klein, MSE

We trust the following compendium will be useful to readers. Chapter 3 of the Compendium is particularly relevant to the design and construction of health care facilities.

Chapter 1   NFPA: What It Is and How It Functions

1-1. Brief History.

The National Fire Protection Association (NFPA) is an independent, voluntary membership, non-profit (tax-exempt) organization. It was formed by insurance underwriters in the Northeast who had been grappling in the late 1800s with the problem of protecting buildings from fire with a new device called an automatic sprinkler. They were finding that the lack of unified rules, or conditions for their installation, was creating confusion. As a result, a group of underwriters met in early 1885 in Boston to explore ways to solve the problem. Subsequent meetings were held in New York City in December of that year, and again in March 1896 to consider sprinkler rules. From these meetings, the group drew up plans for an Association.[1] On November 6, 1896, the National Fire Protection Association was formally established.

The founding officers were all from fire-related insurance companies. How far the Association has come since then in advancing firesafety is difficult to relate in a few short paragraphs. A very detailed and personal account has been written by Percy Bugbee: *Men Against Fire: The Story of the National Fire Protection Association* (Copyright 1971, NFPA Publication No. SPP-14). Mr. Bugbee started working for NFPA in 1921, and was its Chief Executive Officer from 1939 until his retirement in 1968. His book is a glimpse into the files of NFPA from its inception in 1896 up through 1971. It is also a fascinating look at the history of fire as seen by an organization committed to reducing fire losses. It is recommended to both the serious and curious reader.

NFPA has grown from a handful of dedicated insurance under-writers to over 47,000 members from all sectors (see Table D-1); it has developed more than 260 technical documents covering a wide spectrum of firesafety; it supports 225 Technical Commit-tees composed of 4,000 volunteers who produce these docu-ments. The Association has its headquarters in Quincy, Massa-chusetts, where 250 paid staff administer the affairs of the Association. There is a 28-member Board of Directors which oversees the affairs of the Association. NFPA's budget is now over $30 million, financed principally by: (1) membership dues, (2) sales of its publications and audio/visual materials, (3) sponsor-ing of seminars, (4) research grants, and (5) contributions.

In addition to technical documents, NFPA is involved in many different types of educational programs, such as sponsoring Fire Prevention Week each year, holding two Association meetings each year, investigating and reporting on significant fires, and developing a Learn Not to Burn® curriculum for schools.

From one problem (sprinkler standardization), NFPA is now involved in a myriad of activities in the pursuit of "moving mankind towards safety from fire."

TABLE D-1. Approximate make-up of NFPA's 47,000+ members

Affiliation	Percent
Fire Service	31.3
Business and Industry	15.4
Health Care Institutions	12.1
Insurance Companies	7.1
Architects and Engineers	9.0
Fire Equipment Manufacturers and Distributors	5.1
Government	8.1
Education Institutions	3.1
Trade and Professional Associations	2.2
Other	6.6

1-2. Present Staff/Organization.

How does NFPA carry out its mission? Figure D-1 shows how NFPA is organized (both the paid staff and the volunteers) and where the responsibility for services and activities lies.

NFPA is a diversified, multi-dimensional organization (e.g., publisher, sponsor, film producer, investigator, etc.). This is why NFPA is viewed in many different ways by the general public.

1-3. Life Cycle of an NFPA Document.

NFPA has set up a comprehensive procedure for adopting a document. This process has slowly evolved since December 1895, when the group of inspectors met in New York to develop some rules on sprinkler systems. (See Section 1-1 for details.) Today, a complex set of rules called the "Regulations Governing Committee Projects"[2] describes in detail how a project can be created, how it is to be developed, and how resulting documents are to be adopted in order to be published as NFPA codes, standards, manuals, guides, or recommended practices.

All NFPA documents start as Committee Projects. For example: a "problem," brought to the attention of NFPA's Standards Council (a Committee under the Board of Directors), is reviewed and, if considered serious, is given public notice with a request for comments on need, scope, extent of hazard, solutions, etc. If the Council determines there is a sufficient fire or explosion hazard involved, the "problem" will be assigned to an existing NFPA Technical Committee if it is within that Committee's scope, or the Council will set up a new project and appoint a new Committee for the project. It is then up to that Committee to develop the document or documents it believes best solves the "problem" and to present such document(s) for adoption at an NFPA Meeting.

Technical Committees under these "Regulations" are guided by a principle of balanced interests with the criteria that no one interest group compose more than one-third of the Committee, and a wide range of interests are represented. Additionally, since the maximum workable size of a productive Committee is about 25 members, the Standards Council, the group authorized by the NFPA Board of Directors to act on its behalf in the area of standards development, has a tough but critical task fulfilling these criteria in overseeing Technical Committee membership. (The

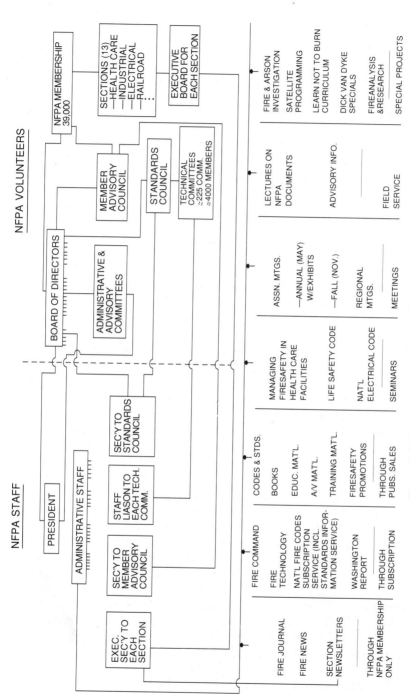

Figure D-1. How NFPA delivers firesafety in the 1980s.

167

Council approves *all* appointments to Technical Committees.) To appreciate the results of this responsibility, readers are referred to the beginning of any NFPA standard, code, etc., where Committee membership at the time of balloting is listed. The names therein did not get included there by chance—it was very deliberate.

The starting point for a new document, or the revision of an existing one, is the formal "call for proposals" period. While proposals for existing documents are accepted anytime, an official time period is set and publicized in order to set in motion all the activities that need to take place to present a document for approval at a particular Association Meeting (Annual or Fall). During the proposal period, all portions of an existing document are open to suggestion, and ideas for the scope and content of new documents are sought. (See Figure D-2(a), Public Proposal Form.) All proposals (those received since the last edition of the document and during the call for proposals period) are then reviewed by the responsible Technical Committee. Action is taken either to accept the proposal, reject it, or accept it in principle (action other than accepting a proposal requires an explanatory statement by the Committee). The Committee may also produce Committee proposals during this time. Accepted and amended proposals thus constitute the Committee's report for a proposed new or revised document.

All proposals for documents reporting to a particular Assn. Meeting (e.g., 1988 Annual Meeting) are then published in a document title *"Technical Committee Reports"* (TCR) . Following this, there is a public comment period (about 80 days) during which time comments can be made on proposals. (NOTE: for a new document, the whole document would be open for public comment.) After the public comment period, Technical Committees take action (similar to that on public proposals) on any public comments submitted. The actions taken on these public comments are then published in a document titled *"Technical Committee Documentation"* (TCD) which, in essence, amends the proposed *Technical Committee Reports*. These two efforts, the TCR and TCD, constitute what is presented for approval at an Association Meeting. And after Assn action, the Standards Council reviews the entire process and, if there are no problems, releases the new or revised documents.

The above overview is very simple, but the process is not, as attested by the 18-month span required to accomplish it. A calendar of events is presented in Figure D-2(b) to help readers grasp

FORM FOR PROPOSALS ON NFPA TECHNICAL COMMITTEE DOCUMENTS

Mail To: Secretary, Standards Council
         National Fire Protection Association, Batterymarch Park,
         Quincy, Massachusetts 02269

Date _____ Name _____ Tel. No. _____

Address _____

Representing (Please indicate organization, company or self)

1. a) Document Title: _____ NFPA No. & Year _____

   b) Section/Paragraph: _____

2. Proposal recommends: (Check one) ☐ new text
                                 ☐ revised text
                                 ☐ deleted text

3. Proposal (include proposed new or revised wording, or identification of wording to be deleted):

4. Statement of Problem and Substantiation for Proposal:

5. ☐ This Proposal is original material.
   ☐ This Proposal is not original material; its source (if known) is as follows: _____

_____

(Note: Original material is considered to be the submitter's own idea based on or as a result of his own
experience, thought, or research and, to the best of his knowledge, is not copied from another source.)

I agree to give NFPA all and full rights, including rights of copyright, in this Proposal and I
understand that I acquire no rights in any publication of NFPA in which this Proposal in this or
another similar or analogous form is used.

_____
                                    Signature

PLEASE USE SEPARATE FORM FOR EACH PROPOSAL

Figure D-2(a). Form for proposals on NFPA Technical Committee documents.

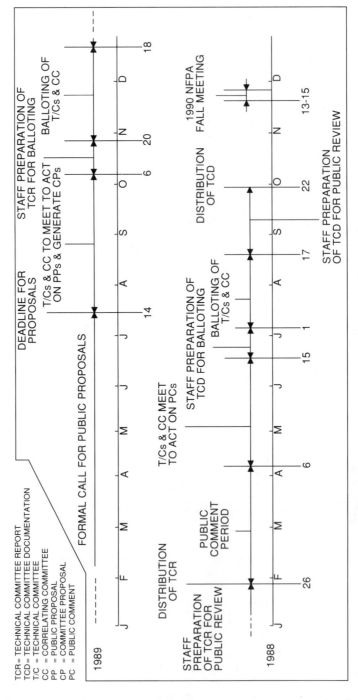

Figure D-2(b). Revision process for documents reporting at an NFPA fall meeting.

TCR = TECHNICAL COMMITTEE REPORT
TCD = TECHNICAL COMMITTEE DOCUMENTATION
T/C = TECHNICAL COMMITTEE
CC = CORRELATING COMMITTEE
PP = PUBLIC PROPOSAL
CP = COMMITTEE PROPOSAL
PC = PUBLIC COMMENT

the complexity of the system necessary to produce NFPA documents.

No one segment of this process should be viewed as a separate entity, for each contributes to achieving consensus and producing a document that will benefit the cause of firesafety. Although not perfect, this system is a good example of how far a voluntary organization can go in seeking and addressing input from as many contributors as possible.

NFPA produces only voluntary standards and codes representing a detailed history of the changes in fire prevention technology. But many of these documents are considered referenced requirements by a variety of authorities having jurisdiction throughout the United States and the world. And it should be noted that development of these standards is accomplished without taxpayer money.

Adoption by authorities of NFPA documents attests to the viability of the NFPA standards-making system. However, since NFPA documents are anything but static, adoption has not been without some problems. At minimum, NFPA documents are reviewed at least once every five years, and very few pass through the system without any changes. As more knowledge in fire technology is gained, materials dealing with the subject must be changed accordingly. But, while NFPA progresses, not all authorities do the same, or at least not at the same pace. Thus, different editions of a document may be adopted by different enforcing authorities at any one time, a situation which may result in confusion for users in both the health care community and in other fields. However, this is not a problem that can or will be solved by NFPA alone. Since the life cycle of a document is one of continual improvements, NFPA would be remiss for not regularly upgrading its products. The problem, therefore, requires a coordinated effort by both the voluntary standards developers and those who utilize such standards.

1-4. NFPA Documents Pertinent to Health Care Facilities.

NFPA publishes about 260 documents in the form of standards, codes, recommended practices, and manuals. The number varies due to withdrawals of dated documents or the adoption of new documents. Not all affect or are intended to affect health care facilities. However, no one sector is affected by all 260 plus documents. Some documents have been developed exclusively for health care facilities (e.g., those dealing with the use of inhalation anesthetics, or health care emergency preparedness). Others, however, affect health care facilities in that a particular function they address may apply to any facility (e.g., sprinkler system installation). In between are documents (e.g., the National Electrical Code® and the Life Safety Code®) that are general in scope but identify different types of facilities and set requirements accordingly because general statements would not cover all situations satisfactorily.

To help health care personnel gain some perspective of the variety of firesafety-related documents that may be utilized before and while a health care facility is occupied (and even after it is no longer occupied), a listing of all the NFPA documents cited in this Compendium is included in Appendix D of this Compendium.

This listing in Appendix D of this Compendium is not meant to imply that health care personnel should ignore the other 180 plus documents not listed. In this age of specialization, tunnelvision is a hazard in and of itself, and anyone seriously interested in firesafety should be aware of to what is being done in other sectors to determine if it has some applicability to his or her own area of interest. NFPA and the public both benefit from the combined expertise of many individuals reviewing documents and submitting comments on them. Hence, health care personnel, while concentrating on firesafety information as it relates to their institutions, should also review other documents as much as possible in order to share their knowledge on firesafety.

1-5. NFPA Health Care Facilities Committee.

As mentioned in Section 1-3, the NFPA Standards Council does not create standards or codes first and then form Committees. The Council first creates a Committee project as a result of a need to address a subject. A Committee is then formed which decides how best to address the subject (e.g., by generating a code, a standard, or a manual).

In the early 1940s, a Committee on Hospitals was established to address the hazards associated with the use of flammable anesthetics in operating rooms. Explosions as a result of using flammable anesthetics were occurring at a rate considered unacceptable. Following the development of guidelines for the use of flammable anesthetics (the application of which reduced both the number of incidents and the potential for them), the Committee began to consider other fire-related hazardous conditions in hospitals and other health care facilities. As a result, a series of documents was developed (the NFPA 56 series and 76 series documents and NFPA 3M). In doing so, the Hospital Committee activities became so extensive that permanent Subcommittees were formed. In 1975, Subcommittees were raised to full Technical Committee status and the Committee on Hospitals became the Health Care Facilities Correlating Committee.

In June 1981, the Standards Council approved a proposal by the Correlating Committee to integrate all the previous individual documents developed by each Committee into one standard. As stated by the Correlating Committee in its request to the Council, the integration was considered necessary for the following reasons:

1. All the health care facilities documents were being revised independently of each other. As a result, it was not always easy to know whether one had the latest edition of a particular document. The proposed new standard, in combining all the documents into one standard, would eliminate this problem.

2. A very significant cost savings was projected for purchasers of the new standard, which would be less expensive to purchase than each of the individual documents. In addition, the Correlating Committee considered the benefits to NFPA, and how production time and money would be saved by printing the 12 separate documents as one bound standard.

3. The integration would place into one unit (of approximately 200 pages) many documents which referenced each other.

4. The Correlating Committee felt that the integration would be an easier and more complete reference for the various users of the documents (e.g., hospital engineers, medical personnel, designers and architects, as well as the various types of enforcing authorities).

The new document, designated NFPA 99, *Standard for Health Care Facilities*, was first published in January 1982 as a compilation of the then 12 individual documents that were under the jurisdiction of the Correlating Committee. Formal adoption of

NFPA 99 occurred at the NFPA 1983 Fall Meeting after following established procedures outlined previously in this Chapter. For 1987, NFPA 99 was completely restructured and made an integrated document. One more document, NFPA 56F, Standard for Nonflammable Medical Piped Gas Systems, was integrated as well into NFPA 99-1987. In addition, and as a result of restructuring, the Health Care Facilities Committee Structure was reorganized: the Correlating Committee was replaced by a new balanced Technical Committee, and the former Technical Committees replaced by new standing Subcommittees. For reference purposes, the new Technical Committee and its scope, and the Subcommittees and their responsibilities, are printed in Table D-2.

NFPA 99 will be revised periodically, again in accordance with NFPA procedures.

TABLE D-2. Current scope of health care facilities technical committee; responsibilities of standing subcommittees

Technical Committtee

Scope: This Committee shall have primary responsibility for developing documents which contain criteria for safeguarding patients and health care personnel in the delivery of health care services within health care facilities:

a) from fire, explosion, electrical and related hazards resulting either from the use of anesthetic agents, medical gas equipment, electrical apparatus and high frequency electricity, or from internal or external incidents that disrupt normal patient care;

b) from fire and explosion hazards associated with laboratory practices;

c) in connection with the use of hyperbaric and hypobaric facilities for medical purposes;

d) through performance, maintenance, and testing criteria for electrical systems, both normal and essential; and

e) through performance, maintenance, testing and installation criteria 1) for vacuum systems for medical or surgical purposes, and 2) for medical gas systems.

Standing Subcommittees	Assignment: (Ref: NFPA 99-1987)
a. Anesthesia Services	Sections 12-4.1 and 13-4.1 (Anesthetizing Locations)

TABLE D-2.—(*Continued*)

b. Disaster Planning	Annex 1 (Health Care Emergency Preparedness)
c. Electrical Systems	Chapter 3 (Electrical Systems) '-3.3' in Chaps 12 to 18
e. Gas Equipment	Chapter 8 (Gas Equipment); '-3.8' in Chaps 12 to 18
f. Hyperbaric & Hypobaric Facilities	Chapter 19 (Hyberbaric Facilities); NFPA 99B, Std. for Hypobrbic Facilities*
g. Laboratories	Chapter 10 (Laboratories)
h. Nonflammable Medical Piped Gas Systems	Gas System Portion of Chapter 4 (Gas & Vacuum Systems); '-3.4' in Chaps. 12 to 18 (gas system portion)
i. Vacuum Systems and Equipment	Vacuum System Portion of Chapter 4 (Gas and Vacuum Systems); '-3.4' in Chaps. 12 to 18 (vacuum system portion)
j. Use of High Frequency Electricity	Annex 2 (Safe Use of High Frequency Electricity in Health Care Facilities)

*Through Technical Committee

Chapter 2   Some Common Terms

In most NFPA technical documents—and most scientific papers —a section is usually included that defines terms to be used throughout the text, especially where it is desired that there be no question as to the intended meaning of a word. While this *Compendium* is not a technical document, a few of the more common terms associated with NFPA documents or related to firesafety are listed below to help readers who may not be familiar with them. (Terms already defined by NFPA are in quotation marks.)

2-1. Types of Technical Documents.

NFPA Committees produced four types of technical documents: manuals, recommended practices, standards, and codes.

Manual (or Guide): "A Document which is informative in nature and does not contain requirements." (NFPA) It is more than what most would term a "report." It offers guidance on a particular fire hazard, and may contain some sources of action for consideration. However, a manual is intentionally not written in a form that an enforcing authority would adopt or require someone within its jurisdiction to comply with.

Recommended Practice: "A Document containing only advisory provisions (using the word 'should' to indicate recommendations) in the body of the text." (NFPA) This type of document is the one most often *not* used as intended. The recommendations contained in the document are only recommendations; they may or may not be the best or only way to address the subject. They are suggested ways—hence the use of the word "should." However, extrapolation of "should" into "shall" has been known to occur, thereby turning suggestions into standards. Government authorities (federal, state, local) are bound by law to adopt only standards. (NFPA recognized this a few years ago, and has arranged its *National Fire Codes* so that only codes and standards are included in Volumes 1-8, and only recommended practices and manuals are included in Volumes 9 through 11.) Unfortunately, non-governmental organizations are not bound by this restriction. It is not the intent of NFPA that recommended practices be adopted. Recommended practices are only recommendations, and should be accepted and used as such.

Standard: "A Document containing only mandatory provisions using the word 'shall' to indicate requirements. Explanatory material may be included only in the form of 'fine print' notes, in footnotes, or in an appendix." (NFPA) Here the Technical Committee makes a technical judgment that the problem is of a sufficient hazard that minimum performance levels or installation requirements are needed, and so states them in definitive or measurable terms.

Code: "A Document containing only mandatory provisions using the word 'shall' to indicate requirements and in a form generally suitable for adoption into law. Explanatory material may be included only in the form of 'fine print' notes, in footnotes, or in an appendix." (NFPA) Here, the Technical Committee has gone one step further than a standard and structured the document in such a way as to make its adoption, if desired by governmental agencies, more expeditious. Other than that, codes and standards are essentially of the same character.

2-2. Standards.

There are several types of standards. A few of the more common types are listed below. Each is developed for a different purpose.

Voluntary Standards: These are standards that are developed and meant to be used voluntarily. As such, they are not binding on any person, company, organization, or institution. It is intended that they serve as a unifying function while at the same time not stifle innovation. They are indicative that a level of development has been reached on a particular subject that allows for some standardization. As should be obvious, when a voluntary standard is utilized by some enforcing authority, the contents of the standard do not change, but its application does.

Manufacturing Standards: These are standards which are measurement related; that is, the item or process described in the standard can be translated into a product with uniformity (e.g., a No. 10 nail or No. 10 screw or a No. 10 envelope can be made by anyone using the appropriate standard with reasonable assurance that it will be the same size or shape as an existing one).

Performance Standards: These are standards that list criteria of integrity but do not stipulate how this integrity is to be achieved (e.g., the door shall be capable of withstanding burning for 1 hour; the power shall be restored within 10 seconds).

Installation Standards: These are standards that detail how a product or material is to be installed or function. They are the result of experience or testing (e.g., No. 10 wire shall be used for grounding purposes).

2-3. Terms Used During the Revision Cycle.

When a document is revised, or a new document is developed by NFPA, it passes through several stages before being approved (as outlined in Chapter 1). Some of the more common terms used during that process are the following:

Public proposal: A written idea or recommendation submittable by anyone at any time on any portion of an existing document. It can also consist of ideas or recommendations for a proposed new document. (See Figure D-2(a) for form used to submit a proposal.)

Committee proposal: A proposal generated by the Technical Committee responsible for the document being revised or the new document being proposed.

Technical Committee Reports (TCR): The results of actions on all proposals by the Technical Committee responsible for the document. The TCR constitutes the revisions or recommendations acceptable to the Committee (i.e., acceptable to at least two-thirds of the Committee). TCR's are distributed to the public for an approximately 80-day public review period.

Public comments: Recommended changes to the TCR that are submitted during the public review period. They are actually comments on proposals, with the only limitation being that the comment must be on the material included in the proposal. Anyone, including Technical Committee members and persons whose proposals were not accepted, can submit public comments. Public comments are acceptable on any portion of a proposed new document since the new document would not have been available to the public during the public proposal period. (This occurs because one proposal is a Committee-generated one that proposes the new document.)

Technical Committee Documentation (TCD): The result of action on all public comments to the TCR by the Technical Committee responsible for the document. The TCD constitutes amendments to the TCR that are acceptable to the Committee (again, through balloting, at least two-thirds of the Committee must be in favor of any amendment). It is the TCR, as amended by the TCD, which is presented to the Association for voting at an Association Meeting. (If no public comments are received, only the TCR is presented for approval.)

Technical Report Session: This is the portion of an NFPA Meeting during which NFPA members attending the Meeting vote on the TCR (as amended by the TCD). Currently, the Association can take the following actions on a Committee Report:

1. Accept it as is.

2. Return the entire Report back to the Committee (i.e., reject it).

3. Return a portion of the Report back to the Committee (thus accepting the other portions).

4. Amend the Report by accepting previously rejected proposals or comments.

Association action is by simple majority of those present.
For actions number 3 and 4, the Technical Committee respon-

sible for the Report is also balloted, with several different results possible depending on whether the Committee upholds by a two-thirds majority the action of the Association Meeting. All Reports, together with Association Meeting recommendations and Technical Committee balloting, are then reviewed by the NFPA Standards Council which has the authority of the NFPA Board of Directors to issue documents.

Complaint: "Any request in writing for a reversal or modification of any action taken by any Committee at any time in the document development process." (NFPA) Complaints are heard by the NFPA Standards Council. A new or revised document is not released until any and all complaints are ajudicated.

Appeal: "Any request in writing for a reversal or modification of any action by the [NFPA] Standards Council taken at any time in the standards development process." (NFPA) Generally an appeal is not requested until all other avenues of change have been exhausted (e.g., if the problem develops during the proposal period, submission of a public comment can be considered). Appeals are heard by the NFPA Board of Directors. (NOTE: No member of the Board of Directors serves on the Standards Council.)

2-4. Consensus.

There are many variations in the definition for this term. NFPA uses the term to denote the *entire process* by which a technical document is revised or promulgated. It starts with the first notice of intent to revise an existing document or propose a new one (i.e., calling for proposals), and continues through the NFPA Standards Council review following Association action. It attempts to take into account the views of the public, of the Technical Committee, and of NFPA members. It is hoped that by this process all persons interested in or knowledgeable on a particular subject will have voiced their concerns at some point so that they may be addressed.

Is NFPA's consensus process perfect? No—but it is considered by many to be the most openly structured and accessible method in the United States for producing a reasonable technical document.

2-5. Terms Related to the Use of NFPA Documents.

NFPA's technical documents are used by consumers, manufacturers, testing laboratories, the government, non-government organizations, and others. In order to promote uniformity of interpretation by such a wide range of users, NFPA has defined the following terms.

Authority Having Jurisdiction: This term refers to that authority which has jurisdiction over an institution, or portion thereof, and which approves some aspects of the institution's operation. The authority can be a federal, state, or local government agency, or it can be some non-government organization (i.e., the Joint Commission on Accreditation of Hospitals, an insurance company, or almost any person or organization who can or does enforce some requirement). (For complete text of definition, see NFPA "Regulations Governing Committee Projects.")

Approved/Labeled/Listed: These terms are fully explained in NFPA "Regulations Governing Committee Projects," and are reprinted below. As noted in these definitions, NFPA does not test, certify, or approve products, installations, etc. Further it is the authority having jurisdiction who determines whether a product, etc. is acceptable. Reference standards such as those developed by NFPA can be and are used. When there is a difference of opinion between parties over the meaning of text within an NFPA standard, NFPA will, upon request, provide an interpretation on the intent of a requirement.

Approved: Acceptable to the "authority having jurisdiction."

NOTE: The National Fire Protection Association does not approve, inspect, or certify any installations, procedures, equipment, or materials nor does it approve or evaluate testing laboratories. In determining the acceptability of installations or procedures, equipment or materials, the "authority having jurisdiction" may base acceptance on compliance with NFPA or other appropriate standards. In the absence of such standards, said authority may require evidence of proper installation, procedure, or use. The "authority having jurisdiction" may also refer to the listings or labeling practices of an organization concerned with product evaluations which is in a position to determine compliance with appropriate standards for the current production of listed items.

Labeled: Equipment or materials to which has been attached a label, symbol, or other identifying mark of an organization acceptable to the "authority having jurisdiction" and concerned with product evaluation, that maintains periodic inspection of production of labeled equipment or materials and by whose labeling the manufacturer indicates compliance with appropriate standards or performance in a specified manner.

Listed: Equipment or materials included in a list published by an organization acceptable to the "authórity having jurisdiction" and concerned with product evaluation, that maintains periodic inspection of production of listed equipment or materials and whose listing states either that the equipment or material meets approprite standards or has been tested and found suitable for use in a specified manner.

> **NOTE:** The means for identifying listed equipment may vary for each organization concerned with product evaluation, some of which do not recognize equipment as listed unless it is also labeled. The "authority having jurisdiction" should utilize the system employed by the listing organization to identify a listed product.

2-6. Fire and Prevention.

It seems appropriate to include a few of the more common — though many times misused — terms related to fire and the ways it is contained or prevented.

2-6.1 Fire.

Fire Load: This is "the expected maximum of combustible material in a given fire area," usually expressed as weight of combustible material per square foot. (NFPA)

Flashover: This is a phenomenon that occurs in a burning room, believed to be caused by thermal radiation feedback from the ceiling and upper parts of walls. When all the combustibles in the space have become heated to their ignition temperatures, ignition takes place simultaneously and rather dramatically.

2-6.2. Fire Prevention.

Fire Resistive: The property or design of a material or structure that enables it to resist the effects of any fire. There are various degrees of fire resistiveness.

Fire Retardant: A lower degree of fire resistance than fire resistive. Here the material or structure is often combustible in whole or part but treated or surface-coated to retard ignition or spread of fire.

Flameproof: This term is not used anymore, as the word can be misleading.

Flame Resistant: This term is used but not approved by NFPA.

Flame Retardant: The chemically treated or inherent properties of material which will not ignite or propagate flames when subjected to a small or moderate fire.

2-7. Safety.

Finally, there is the question of how safe the use of an NFPA document makes an institution, product, or installation (i.e., what is the definition of safe?). There is no simple answer, for part of the answer lies in what people will accept as safe. Nothing is 100 percent safe. What may be more important to ask is what level of safety is *possible* and what level is *acceptable*, given the technology, resources, personnel, and money available, and the severity of the hazard involved. Ideally, the second level (acceptable) can meet the first level (possible); realistically, this is not always the case.

NFPA Technical Committees are aware of the interrelationship of these safety factors, and must make value judgments as to what level of safety, in their opinion, should be obtained. It is not an easy task.

A good analysis of this subject can be found in Chapter 2 of *Standards of Development in the Private Sector: Thoughts on Interest Representation and Procedural Fairness* by Robert G. Dixon, Jr. (Copyright 1978, NFPA.)

Chapter 3   Facility Fire Protection

In expanding on Section 1-4, NFPA Documents Pertinent to Health Care Facilities, a systems approach will be used to indicate where firesafety protection, information, etc., can be found. External facility protection is presented first, with an orderly progression to internal provisions and features. Omission of a subject does not mean that health care facilities should ignore it; rather, it should encourage readers who feel a particular subject

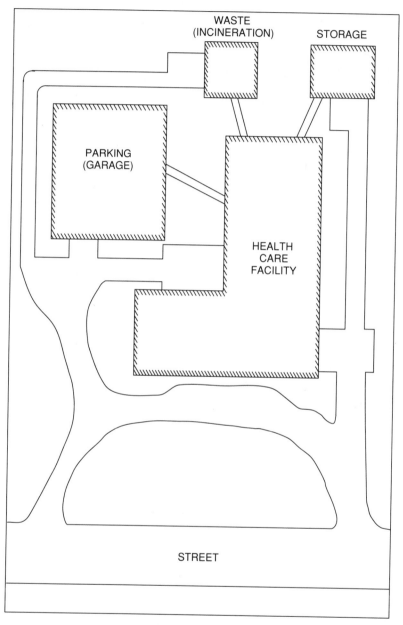

WASTE
(INCINERATION)

STORAGE

PARKING
(GARAGE)

HEALTH
CARE
FACILITY

STREET

Figure D-3. A Health care facility.

or area should have been included to bring it to the attention of the author for incorporation into the next edition of this *Compendium.*

In this chapter, fire protection systems that are built-in will be discussed. These systems are set in place and require little or no human intervention in order to function. (They can require maintenance to continue functioning.) In Chapters 4 and 5, fire protection involving human awareness or intervention will be discussed.

Several areas and structures that pose a fire hazard can be found around many health care facilities. They may or may not be physically attached to the main or central medical portion of the health care facility. These areas or structures include the following.

3-1.1. Parking Garages.

Space limitations often necessitate vertical parking structures of 2, 3, or even 10 or more stories. NFPA 88A-1985, *Standard for Parking Structures*, provides guidance on construction, lighting, heating, ventilation, and detection and fire extinguishment systems for all types of parking garages.

3-1.2. Outdoor or bulk storage of flammable or nonflammable (but oxidizing) gases or liquids is often necessary. Storage may be remote from or adjacent to buildings, and requirements vary accordingly. NFPA has several documents covering this subject. For health care facilities, the more relevant are: NFPA 50-1985, *Standard for Bulk Oxygen Systems at Consumer Sites;* NFPA 58-1986, *Standard for the Storage and Handling of Liquefied Petroleum Gases;* and NFPA 30-1987, *Flammable and Combustible Liquids Code.*

NFPA 50 lists the various distances at which bulk oxygen systems should be located from parked vehicles, places of assembly, etc. It also includes system fabrication requirements.

NFPA 58 lists design, construction, installation, and operation guidance for liquefied petroleum gases, including various types of installations (e.g., roofs, remote, vehicular).

NFPA 30 covers a wide spectrum of requirements on the storage and use of flammable and combustible liquids. Chapter 4 of NFPA 30 includes guidance on outdoor storage of containers and portable tanks.

3-1.3. Hydrants and External Water Supplies.

It is not possible for fire service personnel to carry sufficient water for all situations. Thus, they must rely on external sources, such as hydrants. The location, pressure, and supply rate are usually specified by local fire prevention codes. These factors are considered when initially locating a health care facility.

The Insurance Services Office (60 Water St., New York, NY 10038) publishes material on hydrant flow requirements.

Large reservoirs (tanks) of water are sometimes built, when necessary, expressly for sprinkler or standpipe systems. NFPA has developed a document on tanks used for that purpose, NFPA 22-1984, *Standard for Water Tanks for Private Fire Protection*. It offers guidance on the design, construction, installation, and maintenance of the various types of tanks employed (steel gravity, wood gravity, embankment-supported rubberized fabric, steel tower) as well as ancillary equipment (pipe connections) and guidance on protection against freezing.

A general discussion of water supplies is included in the NFPA *Fire Protection Handbook*, 16th Edition (Section 17, Chapters 3, 4, 5, and 8).

NFPA also publishes a standard—NFPA 24-1984, *Standard for Private Fire Service Mains and Their Appurtenances*—which provides guidance on outdoor underground piping for fire extinguishing purposes (Chapters 1 and 8); guidance on water supplies and hydrant locations (Chapters 2 and 4); and guidance on fire department connections for standpipe and sprinkler systems (Chapter 2, Section 2-6).

3-1.4. Fire Lanes.

Access to buildings by fire department vehicles is esssential. Criteria on this subject are listed in Chapter 3 of NFPA 1-1987, *Fire Prevention Code*.

3-1.5. Disposal and Incinerators.

Disposal of waste products, both hazardous and non-hazardous, continues to draw increasing attention, not only because of environmental considerations but also because of the sheer amounts being generated. The Environmental Protection Agency has issued regulations on the disposal of hazardous waste, and health care facilities are not exempt from these regulations. For details, readers should contact the Environmental Protection Agency, Washington, D.C. 20460.

NFPA has developed a document on incinerators, NFPA 82-1983, *Standard on Incinerators, Waste and Linen Handling Systems and Equipment.* Guidance on design, placement, clearances, etc., is included in Chapter 2. In addition, the NFPA *Fire Protection Handbook* (16th Edition) includes information on incinerators in Section 12, Chapter 15.

3-1.6. Location of Structure.

The site of a building in relation to other buildings also has to be considered (e.g., how a fire in a nearby building would affect the health care facility's building(s)). To that end, NFPA has developed a document, NFPA 80A-1987, *Recommended Practice for Protection of Buildings from Exterior Fire Exposures.* It provides recommended separation distances between buildings; means of protection between buildings; and methods of reducing separation distances.

3-2. Life Safety Consideratioins for Health Care Facilities.

The ability of occupants to leave a building in a fire emergency is one of the prime concerns of NFPA *101r®-1985, Life Safety Code* (Full Title: *Code for Safety to Life from Fire in Buildings and Structures*). This document originated in 1913 following a growing problem of exiting from high-rise buildings in a fire emergency. The document now covers a host of topics, though all are related to the problem of reducing the spread of fire in a building, and providing means of egress from a building should it become necessary in a fire situation. The *Life Safety Code* recognizes the need for different requirements for different types of occupancies (hotels, home, hospital, etc.) and makes provisions accordingly.

3-2.1. General requirements on *exiting* are contained in Chapter 5 of the 1985 edition of NFPA *101*; Chapters 12 and 13 include specific requirements for health care facilities (12-2 and 13-2, respectively). The three major components of exiting (the official term is means of egress) are:

1. Exit Access: Those portions of a means of egress (such as a corridor, an aisle) which lead to an entrance to an exit.

2. Exit: That portion of a means of egress that is separated from all other spaces of a building by construction and thus provides a protected way of travel to the exit discharge. The exit includes the exit door(s), protected stairways, and landings.

3. Exit Discharge: That portion of a means of egress between the end of the "exit" and a public way (such as a sidewalk open to outside air).

An excellent discussion on the concept of egress design (exiting), including psychological as well as physiological factors, is included in the NFPA *Fire Protection Handbook* (16th Edition) (Section 7, Chapter 3).

Laboratories need some special requirements for exiting because of the nature of activities therein. Section 10-3.2 of NFPA 99-1987, *Standard for Health Care Facilities*, provides additional requirements for exiting from laboratories.

3-2.2. The three other major areas covered by NFPA *101* are: *construction features* requirements in Chapter 6 (e.g., smoke barriers, interior finish); *building service and fire protection* requirements in Chapter 7 (e.g., utilities, heating, air conditioning, smoke control, elevators, rubbish chutes, detection systems, fire extinguishment systems); and *operating features* for each type of occupancy (e.g., furnishings, fire exit drills) in Chapter 31.

3-2.3. Specific life safety requirements for health care facilities are covered in Chapter 12 (new occupancies) and Chapter 13 (existing occupancies) of NFPA *101*. Extensive commentary on life safety requirements for health care occupancies can also be found in Section 9, Chapter 4 of the NFPA *Fire Protection Handbook* (16th Edition).

3-3. Structural Protection.

Firesafety considerations for the structural portion of a health care facility building are essentially the same as for other buildings. However, the requirements for these structural portions in health care facilities may differ from those for other types of occupancies. Thus, readers are cautioned to review carefully the references provided for any special requirements for health care facilities.

3-3.1. NFPA has developed a code for lightning protection, NFPA 78-1986, *Lightning Protection Code*. It lists configurations, conductors, grounding provisions, etc., that are necessary in providing lightning protection for a building.

3-3.2. The transport of patients by helicopter is increasing. As a result, any consideration of a rooftop helicopter facility should include a review of requirements contained in NFPA 418-1979, *Standard on Rooftop Heliport Construction and Protection*.

3-3.3. A uniform classification scheme for the various types of building construction has also been developed by NFPA. It is contained in NFPA 220-1985, *Standard on Types of Building Construction*. This document classifies exterior bearing walls, interior bearing walls, columns, etc., into five types, depending on (1) the non-combustibility or limited combustibility of the material of the wall, column, etc., and (2) the fire-resistive rating of the material.

3-3.4. Another classification scheme has been developed by NFPA for windows and doors. The document, NFPA 80-1986, *Standard for Fire Doors and Windows*, provides criteria on the "installation and maintenance of fire door assemblies, windows, glass blocks, and shutters for the protection of openings in walls to restrict the spread of fire and smoke within buildings" (from the scope of NFPA 80). The document sets up a classification scheme based on how well a door or window can withstand fire and heat (i.e., performance criteria).

3-3.5. Chimneys, fireplaces, and vents are the subject of NFPA 211-1984, *Standard for Chimneys, Fireplaces, Vents and Solid Fuel Burning Appliances*. It includes guidance relative to the type of chimney for various types of appliances (including incinerators). Installation, clearances, and drafts requirements are among other items included.

3-3.6 The fire-resistive rating for floor-ceiling assemblies, walls used to form compartments, and the flame spread rating of finish materials inside a building are addressed by NFPA *101*-1985, the *Life Safety Code*. The fire-resistivity "time" built into various materials and construction to contain a fire and/or its rate of spread is the time needed by occupants to exit a building. Paragraph 6-2.2.10 of NFPA *101* provides fire-resistive rating criteria for floor assemblies, etc., referencing NFPA 251-1985, *Standard Methods of Fire Tests of Building Construction and Materials*. Paragraphs 12-3.6 and 13-3.6 of NFPA *101* list criteria specifically for health care facilities. Section 6-5 of NFPA 101 provides flamespread criteria and classification for interior finish mterials, referencing NFPA 255-1984, *Methods of Test of Surface Burning Characteristics of Building Materials*. Paragraphs 12-3.3 and 13-3.3 of NFPA *101* list criteria specifically for health care facilities.

By knowing such things as the different flame and smoke characteristics of material, and how much heat a particular method of construction can withstand, architects, engineers, etc., can make the necessary calculations in the design stage of a building to meet firesafety requirements.

3.3-7. Again, laboratories have some unique operations requiring special considerations with regard to structural fire protection. Sections 10-3.1 and 10-3.2 of NFPA 99-1987, *Standard for Health Care Facilities*, provide criteria on construction, exit details, and fire protection for laboratories. The NFPA *Fire Protection Handbook* (16th Edition) also contains information on laboratory protection (see Section 12, Chapter 2 of the *Handbook*).

3-4. Detection and Extinguishment Systems.

To help reduce detection time, methods of detecting smoke, heat, and fire, etc., have been developed. In addition, systems that can suppress and extinguish a fire (either manually or automatically) can be installed to reduce the amount of time before human activity would or could begin to extinguish a fire.

Detection and extinguishment systems are grouped together here because of their integration in many installations.

3-4.1. Detection Systems.

Standardization of, and standards for, fire detection systems have evolved over the years in conjunction with NFPA *101*-1985, *Life Safety Code*. NFPA 101 states, within a structure, what portion(s) and/or under what circumstances fire, heat, or smoke must be monitored. For new health care facilities, requirements are listed in 12-3.4 of NFPA *101*; for existing facilities, requirements are listed in 13-3.4. Other NFPA Committees have developed documents classifying detectors of fire, heat, or smoke, as well as provided guidance on their performance and installation. Enforcement authorities thus have a uniform reference when deciding what detector(s) would be suitable in a particular application.

Fire detection systems can be viewed as consisting of two parts: (1) the detector portion and (2) the control/indicating portion (see Figure D-4).

(1) Detector Portion.

Detectors do what their name implies — detect something. In firesafety, this can mean sensing (detecting) heat, smoke, flame, gas, or anything else that indicates a fire or explosion is in the making. NFPA has developed two standards on detectors: NFPA 72E-1987, *Standard on Automatic Fire Detectors*; and NFPA 74-1984, *Standard for the Installation, Maintenance, and Use of Household Fire Warning Equipment*. (The former can be used by health care facilities; the latter is applicable only within family dwelling units.)

NFPA 72E was developed for those situations where detectors are to be connected together to form a system which would include a control panel for local or distant indication and announcement of detection (discussed below). The document classifies detection based on operating principles and temperature; it also provides criteria on performance for different types of detectors and their modes of operation, and locating, mounting, and testing these detectors. The document must be used on conjunction with other NFPA documents (discussed below).

In Chapter 4, Section 16 of the NFPA *Fire Protection Handbook* (16th Edition), an extensive, illustrated discussion about detectors can be found.

NFPA 74 provides criteria for the selection, installation, operation, and maintenance of fire warning equipment within family living units. Both smoke and heat detectors are covered in the document. In addition, an extensive appendix includes recommendations for locating detectors in typical home arrangements.

Detectors are also built into sprinkler heads of sprinkler sys-

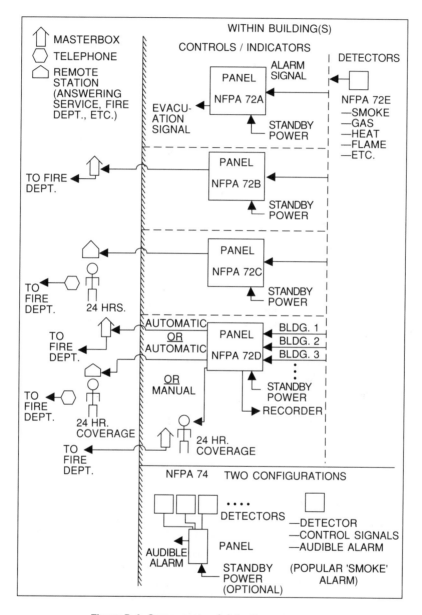

Figure D-4. Components of detection systems.

tems. When the air around these sprinkler heads reaches a particular temperature, pre-set sensors snap, melt, or break, thus allowing water to flow out. Temperature ratings for such detectors are contained in Paragraph 3-16.6 of NFPA 13-1987, *Standard for the Installation of Sprinkler Systems.*

(2) Control/Indicating Portion.

Once a detector senses an environment in excess of a present level (e.g., a set density of smoke, a set temperature, a specific rate of rise in temperature), the condition has to be translated into a form (e.g., a light on a panel, a loud whistle, etc.) that people can recognize in order to take appropriate action. This notification (only) is the way some systems function; others automatically cause something in addition to occur. (For example, NFPA 74 contains requirements for systems that are self-contained or wired together and produce sound automatically within the living unit when the detector senses heat, etc.)

For more complex systems, NFPA has developed a series of documents for each system.

NFPA 72A-1987, *Standard for the Installation, Maintenance and Use of Local Protective Signaling Systems for Guard's Tour, Fire Alarm and Supervisory Service,* provides criteria for those supervised fire detection systems providing fire alarm or supervisory signals within the protected premises. This type of system could include more than just a detector and alarm as outlined in NFPA 74. It could include such features as system trouble signals, evacuation signals for occupants, manual fire alarm boxes located within the premises (though connected only to the system within the premises), guard's tour monitoring, and water-flow alarm monitoring of sprinkler systems.

NFPA 72B-1986, *Standard for the Installation, Maintenance and Use of Auxiliary Protective Signaling Systems for Fire Alarm Service,* provides criteria for the equipment and electrical circuits between the fire detection system within a building and the fire department via a municipal fire alarm system. This type of system provides both detection capability and automatic notification to the fire department. The document includes performance criteria for three types of auxiliary alarm systems and typical wiring diagrams.

NFPA 72C-1986, *Standard for the Installation, Maintenance and Use of Remote Station Protective Signaling Systems,* is similar to NFPA 72B, except that it provides criteria for equipment and electrical circuits that link the fire detection system within a building to a remote station which must be staffed continuously. It is the person at the remote station who takes the appropriate action to initiate fire department response. The method of linking in NFPA 72C, however, can be commercial telephone lines to any location acceptable to the authority having jurisdiction (including, but not limited to, direct linkage to a fire station).

A more complex detector system is one for large buildings or several buildings under one ownership where the fire detection system is under 24-hour supervision. NFPA 72D-1986, *Standard for the Installation, Maintenance and Use of Proprietary Protective Signaling Systems*, includes minimum criteria for the system as well as for operating personnel. This system, like those described in NFPA 72B or 72C, must be linked with one that can transmit the problem to the fire department.

NFPA has also developed a document for large systems that combine the monitoring capabilities included in NFPA 72D and the transmitting capabilities included in NFPA 72B and NFPA 72C. NFPA 71-1987, *Standard for the Installation, Maintenance and Use of Central Station Signaling Systems*, is very similar to an NFPA 72D system except that the central station is privately owned, and buildings owned by various people or companies can be monitored.

For these systems, NFPA recently developed a guideline to test each one. It is NFPA 72H-1984, *Guide for Testing Procedures for Local, Auxiliary, Remote Station and Proprietary Protective Signaling Systems*. It provides recommendations for the maintenance and testing of signaling systems, except for central station signaling systems.

3-4.2. Fire Extinguishment Systems.

Fire extinguishment systems were among the first areas addressed by NFPA when it was formed in 1896. Since then, systems have been refined to a rather exact science of hydraulic calculations and precise location of suppressors (sprinkler heads) for maximum effect. Manual as well as automatic extinguishment systems have been developed and will be discussed in this section.[3]

For purposes of discussion, fire extinguishment systems will be grouped into two types: (1) water, and (2) chemical. Both types are utilized in health care facilities.

(1) Water extinguishment systems can be further divided into sprinkler type and standpipe type. Sprinkler systems consist of a source of water (municipal or stored), piping throughout a building, and precisely spaced sprinklers attached to these pipes near the ceiling of each area. The sprinklers have a thermal sensing part (detector) that snaps, melts, or breaks at some pre-set temperature, thereby allowing water in the pipe to discharge. This is a very simplified description. NFPA 13-1987, *Standard for the Installation of Sprinkler Systems*, provides criteria on the various types of sprinkler systems now in use, and how they are to be activated (i.e., there are wet type, dry type, and deluge type; there are automatically and manually activated types). Included also is guidance for systems in buildings that are located in earthquake-prone areas (see 3-10.3 of NFPA 13). NFPA has also developed a document for maintaining automatic sprinkler systems (NFPA 13A-1981), *Recommended Practice for the Care and Maintenance of Sprinkler Systems*). It outlines important factors to consider for maintaining systems. It also includes owner responsibilities.

The NFPA *Fire Protection Handbook* (16th Edition) devotes an entire section (Section 18) to sprinkler-type extinguishment systems (including fundamentals, types, alarms, and maintenance).

The other type of water extinguishment system is called a standpipe system, and is somewhat similar to the sprinkler type discussed above in that there is need for a source of water and for piping to be connected to the water source throughout the building. However, instead of sprinkler heads, hoses are connected to the pipes (called standpipes) at strategic points throughout a building. NFPA has developed the following documents associated with these systems.

NFPA 14-1986, *Standard for the Installation of Standpipe and Hose Systems*, provides minimum criteria for the installation of these systems (e.g., location and number of standpipes, hose connections, classification of system based on the size of hoses used, types of systems, water supply, and piping).

NFPA 1961–1987, *Standard for Fire Hose*, provides minimum criteria for the various types and sizes of fire hoses in use today. Included are tests such as hydrostatic, pressure, link, burst, etc.

NFPA 1962–1987, *Standard for the Care, Use and Maintenance of Fire Hose*, provides criteria on lined, unlined, and rubber hoses (e.g., inspecting, washing, drying, storing).

In addition, the NFPA *Fire Protection Handbook* (15th Edition) discusses standpipe and hose systems in Chapter 6 of Section 18.

Many water-type extinguishment systems require the use of pump to increase and/or maintain an adequate water pressure in the system, both initially and after the system has activated. There are equations for calculating this pressure. An NFPA Committee was formed in 1899 to address the subject of fire pumps which were then only secondary supplies for water. Today fire pumps are essential for all high-rise buildings as they are the only way to have water reach upper floors with sufficient pressure to have an effect on a fire. Fire pumps also raise the pressure in many other facilities where the water pressure from a tank or municipal supply is not adequate. NFPA 20-1983, *Standard for the Installation of Centrifugal Fire Pumps*, offers criteria on the selection, installation, and maintenance of fire pumps. The various types of pumps now used (electric and diesel; turbine) are discussed.

NFPA 101-1985, *Life Safety Code*, includes requirements for health care facilities with regard to water-type fire suppression systems. New health care facility requirements are listed in 12-3.5 of the document; existing health care facility requirements are listed in 13-3.5.

For the serious reader, other books have been published on water extinguishment systems:

Automatic Sprinklers and Standpipe Systems by Dr. John L. Bryan (Copyright 1976, NFPA) discusses the basic concepts and principles of all types of sprinkler and standpipe systems.

Hydraulics for Fire Protection by Harry E. Hickey, Ph.D., (Copyright 1980, NFPA) is a textbook covering the hydraulics of water used for fire protection.

Hydraulic Institute Standards for Centrifugal, Rotating and Reciprocating Pumps, Hydraulic Institute, 1230 Keith Building, Cleveland, Ohio 44115.

(2) The other major types of extinguishment systems are those employing chemicals (as opposed to water).[4] Of the various types available, three can be seen in health care facilities: carbon dioxide (CO_2), Halon 1301, and dry chemical. For each of these systems, NFPA has developed a standard which covers installation, testing, use, and limitations (i.e., the type(s) of fires which the system was designed to extinguish):

NFPA 12-1985, *Standard on Carbon Dioxide Extinguishing Systems*

NFPA 12A-1985, *Standard on Halon 1301 Fire Extinguishing Systems*

NFPA 17-1985, *Standard on Dry Chemical Extinguishing Systems*

Additional discussion on these systems is included in Section 19 (Chapters 1, 2, and 3, respectively) of the NFPA *Fire Protection Handbook* (16th Edition).

Because of the interest surrounding the use of halogenated extinguishing systems for computer installations, readers may wish to review the following articles in NFPA's *Fire Journal*:[5]

"Testing the Performance of Halon 1301 on Real Computer Installations," R. R. Cholin (Vol. 66, No. 5, September 1972, pp. 105–108).

"Halon 1301 Protection for a Computer Facility," G. W. Bonawitz (Vol. 67, No. 5, September 1973, pp. 134–135).

3-5. Fire Protection for Fixed, Building-Wide Systems (Services).

Within health care facilities, there are systems or services that encompass or connect all or major portions of the structure. Some systems such as heating, cooling, lighting, detecting, communicating, extinguishing, and collecting can be found in other types of occupied structures as well. Others, however, (e.g., piped medical gas systems) are unique to health care facilities. Guidelines have been developed for the fire protection of those that present fire or explosion hazards. These guidelines cover the system itself, and/or the facility as a result of the system's presence, e.g., firesafety criteria during construction or installation; or criteria on the type of separation from other activities during operation).

For purposes of discussion, and ease of reference, these systems or services will be grouped into the following three categories:

- Fire protection for environmental air building service systems (e.g., heating, cooling, exhausting);

- Fire protection for electrical building service systems (e.g., electrical wiring, emergency power);

- Fire protection for specific building service systems (e.g., refuse and laundry chutes, piped gas and vacuum systems).

3-5.1. Fire   Protection   for   Environmental   Air   Building
Service Systems.

Controlling the temperature (and, in many instances today, the
humidity) within a building is a normal part of operating the
building. The elements involved in such a system are either
highly combustible (i.e., the fuels needed to generate heat) or
critical in controlling smoke spread in an emergency (i.e., the
forcing of air throughout the facility by a forced air system). As a
result, NFPA has developed documents that address each area:
(1) fuels; (2) heaters; and (3) airmovers.

(1) Fuels.

Two sources of energy that are often used by health care facilities
and present a fire and explosion hazard are oil and gas.
    Safeguards for the handling of oil when it becomes a health
care facility responsibility (i.e., after it is delivered) are included
in NFPA 30-1987, *Flammable and Combustible Liquids Code.*
Chapter 2 of NFPA 30 provides criteria on tank storage; Chapter 3
covers pipes, valves, and fittings.
    Safeguards in the handling of gas are included in NFPA
54-1984, *National Fuel Gas Code.* Part 2 of NFPA 54 covers gas
piping system design, materials, and components; Part 3 covers
gas piping installations; and Part 4 covers inspection, testing, and
purging.

(2) Heaters.

Devices used to heat a building (either by heating water or air)
require different fire protection considerations, depending on
their size and the fuel utilized. Table D-3 indicates the appropriate document that has been developed for each.
    NFPA 54-1984, *National Fuel Gas Code,* Part 6, provides cri-
teria on the installation of various types of heaters (e.g., central
heating boilers and furnaces; direct make-up air heaters, duct
furnaces, floor furnaces).
    NFPA 31-1987, *Standard for the Installation of Oil Burning
Equipment,* provides minimum requirements for safety to life
and property from fire in the installation of storage tanks, acces-
sories (piping, pumps, valves), and the oil burner itself.
    NFPA 85A-1987, *Standard for Prevention of Furnace Explo-
sions in Fuel Oil- and Natural Gas-Fired Single Burner Boiler
Furnaces,* provides minimum requirements for the design, instal-

TABLE D-3. Fire protection guides for the various types and sizes of building heaters

Fuel	Size		
	Up to approx. 400,000 Btu/hour	Approx. 400,000 Btu/hr to 12.5 million Btu/hour	Approx. 12.5 million Btu/hour and greater
Gas	NFPA 54	ANSI Z83.3	NFPA 85A
Oil	NFPA 31	NFPA 31	NFPA 85A

lation, operation, and maintenance of burners (e.g., the fire box, scrubbers, exhaust) that have a capacity greater than approximately 12.5 million Btu/hour.

ANSI Z82.3, *Standard for Gas Utilization Equipment in Large Boilers,*[6] includes firesafety criteria for those portions of boilers where gas is utilized.

(3) Air Movers.

Movement of air in buildings, whether for heating or cooling, also presents the possibility of moving smoke or facilitating the spread of heat or fire in the event of a fire. NFPA has developed two documents that provide guidance for systems which move air within a building.

For structures less than 25,000 cu ft in volume, NFPA 90B-1984, *Standard for the Installation of Warm Air Heating and Air Conditioning Systems*, is applicable. For larger buildings, NFPA 90A-1985, *Standard for the Installation of Air Conditioning and Ventilating Systems* is applicable. These two documents include provisions for restricting smoke, heat, and fire spread through a duct system in a building; for maintaining building integrity when a duct system is used; and for permitting a duct system to be used for smoke control in an emergency. Each document includes guidance on the entire air system—the heating and cooling equipment, the ducts, the fans, the wiring, building construction integrity, and controls.

3-5.2. Fire Protection for Electrical Building Service Systems.

Electricity is somewhat like the human body's circulatory system: it is a conveyor of energy. By itself, electricity has no meaning; however, it provides the "means" to do an immeasurable number of things in our modern technology age. One side effect of electricity is its fire and shock potential. Uncontrolled, electricity can quickly heat a material so that it will burn or even explode. Additionally, the human body is a reasonably good conductor of electricity, thus presenting a shock hazard if electricity enters the body. In a medical setting, that conductivity is at times enhanced by the very nature of activities performed on a patient. Because of these hazards, NFPA has developed several documents addressing the subject of electricity and safeguarding its use. For health care facilities, these documents cover: (1) installation of wiring; and (2) provision for emergency power.[7]

(1) Installation.

By far, the most comprehensive document on electrical construction and installation is NFPA 70-1987, *National Electrical Code*. This document provides criteria on wiring design, methods, material, and installation, and on associated electrical equipment. Included are specifications for the interconnecting of electrical wiring (e.g., by circuit breakers, outlets, junction boxes), and to portions of electrical equipment, particularly as they interface with the electrical wiring system. Of particular interest to health care personnel is Article 517 of NFPA 70, which is devoted solely to health care facilities.

Article 517[8] contains electrical installation criteria for various types of health care facilities (e.g., clinics, hospitals, nursing homes), as well as for several types of locations within health care facilities (e.g., patient care areas, inhalation anesthetizing locations).[9]

(2) Emergency Electrical Power.

Because of the critical role electrical devices play in the treatment of patients today, and because of the immobility of many patients, continuous electrical power (or power very briefly interrupted, depending upon the procedures involved) is essential for health care facilities. Chapter 3, Electrical Systems, of NFPA 99-1987, *Standard for Health Care Facilities*, provides criteria on (1) the power generator system needed to supply electrical power in the event the normal supply fails; (2) how such a system is to be connected to the normal electrical distribution system, and (3) what circuits, outlets, or functions are to be connected to the system. In Chapters 12 to 18 of NFPA 99, the type and extent of an essential electrical system for various types of health care facilities (e.g., clinics, hospitals, nursing homes, etc.) is listed.

3-5.3. Fire Protection for Specific Building Service Systems.

The third type of building-wide systems consists of those that perform a specific, more limited function than the two types of systems discussed above. These systems are:

1. Piped gas systems.

2. Piped Vacuum Systems.

3. Chutes (e.g., waste, linen).

4. Elevators.

5. Fans (e.g., exhausting).

(1) Piped Gas Systems.

Health care facilities use extensive amounts of both flammable and nonflammable gases. (Note: many of the nonflammable gases will support or enhance combustion.) At some usage level, the installation of a system of pipes to carry the gas (or gases) from a central storage point to various parts of a facility, instead of individual portable cylinders, can be justified both on a safety basis and a financial basis.

The advantages of a piped system for medical gases are a continuous supply of gas available at any time, a lower operating cost, and a lower operating pressure (about 50 psi in pipes as opposed to 2200 psi in cylinders). The disadvantages are the initial cost of installing pipes and the fire and explosion hazards of gases being circulated in pipes throughout a facility. (Note: for the latter similar hazards prevail when many cylinders are present.) To address this problem, NFPA developed a document, NFPA 56F, *Standard for Nonflammable Medical Gas Systems*, (incorporated into the 1987 edition of NFPA 99) which provides general criteria on the installation and testing of systems for piping nonflammable medical gases (e.g., oxygen, medical compressed air, carbon dioxide, helium, etc.), throughout a facility. This includes requirements for the central supply system; monitors and alarms for the system; piping and valves criteria; installation and testing; and guidance for small systems in nonhospital-based facilities. These requirements are contained in Sections 4–3 to 4–6 of NFPA 99-1987, with the type of system to be installed in a particular facility listed in Chapters 12 to 18 of the document.

For laboratories, requirements for piped gas systems are contingent on whether the laboratory is covered under NFPA 99 or NFPA 45.

(a) Laboratories covered by NFPA 99. For nonflammable piped gas systems, requirements are listed in Sections 4-4.3.2, and 4-4.3.7 in NFPA 99-1987. For flammable piped gas systems, requirements are listed in 4-4.3.1, 4-4.3.5, 4-4.3.6 and 4-4.3.8.

(b) Laboratories not covered by NFPA 99. For these laboratories, Chapter 8 of NFPA 45-1986 lists requirements for piped gas systems.

For all other piped gas systems, requirements are contained in NFPA 54-1984, National Fuel Gas Code.

(2) Piped Vacuum Systems

In an opposite sense, a system of pipes can be connected to a central vacuum pump to provide suctioning capability at various points throughout a facility (in lieu of individual suction machines). Some hazards exist with the use of these systems. Section 4-7 to 4-10 of NFPA 99-1987, *Standard for Health Care Facilities*, provides minimum sizing, alarms, installation, maintenance, and testing of a piped vacuum system dedicated for patients use. Chapters 12 to 18 of the document specify the type of vacuum system required for a particular facility.

Finally, Chapter 4, Section 12 of the NFPA *Fire Protection Handbook* (16th Edition) describes some of the hazards associated with gases and with piping gases within a facility, as well as hazards with central vacuum systems.

(3) Chutes.

The installation of chutes in a building is accomplished to reduce the buildup of waste, dirty linen, etc., in patient areas and to eliminate the need for personnel to go around and collect it. However, these installations pose fire hazards in that they cut through smoke barriers, thereby providing a means for fire and smoke to spread if precautions are not taken. While eliminating a buildup of combustibles in one area, they create a buildup of combustibles in another area. Precautions have been developed and are included in NFPA 82-1983, *Standard on Incinerators, Waste and Linen Handling Systems and Equipment*. This document provides criteria for reducing the fire hazards resulting from the installation and use of such chutes, and covers construction criteria, the "chute terminal" room, automatic fire suppression systems, protection for openings through which chutes penetrate, and storage rooms.

In addition, 12-5.4 and 13-5.4 of NFPA 101-1985, *Life Safety Code*, contain criteria specifically for health care facilities with regard to chutes.

(4) Elevators.

Another system that cuts through smoke barriers in a large way is the elevator system. In addition to the fire problems these systems create (which are similar to those of chutes), elevators add the "human load" factor. The American Society of Mechanical Engineers has developed a document that provides criteria on all types of elevators: ANSI/ASME A17.1, *Safety Code for Elevators, Dumb Waiters, Escalators and Moving Walks*.[10]

In addition, 12-5.3 and 13-5.3 of NFPA 101-1985, *Life Safety Code*, contain criteria specifically for health care facilities with regard to elevators, dumb waiters, and vertical conveyors.

(5) Fans.

Removal of certain types of dusts, air, and vapor that are flammable or combustible presents several fire and explosion hazards. They include (1) the substance being removed; (2) the system removing the substance; and (3) the building in which the system is installed. NFPA 91-1983, *Standard for the Installation of Blower and Exhaust Systems for Dust, Stock and Vapor Removal or Conveying*, provides criteria for such systems and includes system design, controls, fans, and fire extinguishment features.

3-6. Fire Protection for Fixed Localized Systems.

A multitude of activities takes place within health care facilities. Some are no different from those occurring in other industries: computer operations; cooking; storing; disposal. Others, however, are unique to health care facilities: surgical procedures; X-rays; treatment clinics. As a result, fixed localized systems of fire protection for these activities have been devised.[11] Again, it is suggested that readers review general documents carefully for any requirements specifically for health care facilities.

For purposes of discussion, fixed localized systems has been divided into two groupings: areas where storage primarily occurs; and areas where some on-going activity is taking place.

3-6.1. Firesafety and Storage.

Firesafety and storage involve several considerations: the combustibility and flammability of the substance being stored; the amount being stored; the type of construction or enclosure for the substance being stored; and the type of supervision or monitoring of the storage area.

NFPA documents providing criteria for the many types of storage that can occur in health care facilities are listed below.

General Storage. General storage criteria of a broad range of combustibles up to 30 ft in height at any one point are included in NFPA 231-1987, *Standard for Indoor General Storage*. In addition to classifying commodities, the document provides criteria on storage arrangement, building construction, fire protection (depending on the type of commodity), and optional safety practices.

Rack Storage. Storage of combustibles on racks could be considered a subgrouping of general storage. However, because of particular hazards associated with this way of storing combustibles, NFPA has developed a document addressing just this subject. NFPA 231C-1986, *Standard for Rack Storage of Materials*, provides criteria in much the same way as NFPA 231.

Historical-Type Data Storage. Since health care facilities must maintain clinical records almost indefinitely, concerns for their long-term safe storage (including protection from fire) are somewhat unique in that to replace the information on these records is virtually impossible. NFPA has developed a manual for this type of storage, NFPA 232AM-1986, *Manual for Fire Protection for Archives and Records Centers*, which, like NFPA 232 (but in manual instead of standard form), gives information on the problems associated with this type of storage. It includes fire risks, programs for fire preventions operations guidelines, and fire control methods, including a comparison between types of methods of detection and suppression. Results of tests run by government and non-government labs are included in a specification for firesafe construction for any archive or record center.

Flammable Liquids Storage. Criteria on the safe indoor storage of flammable liquids are contained in several NFPA documents. General criteria are provided in Chapter 6 of NFPA 30-1987, *Flammable and Combustible Liquids Code*. For specific criteria for health care laboratories, Section 10-7.2 of NFPA 99-1987, *Standard for Health Care Facilities*, should be consulted. Paragraph 7-2.3 of NFPA 45-1986, *Laboratories Using Chemicals*, contains criteria for other laboratories.

Flammable and Nonflammable Medical Gas Storage. Unlike flammable liquids, there is no general document with criteria for flammable gas storage. This is due to the widely different forms in which gas is provided. The NFPA documents developed for the various types of gas storage include the following:

1. For storage of *gas cylinders* used in nonflammable medical piped gas systems, NFPA 99-1987, *Standard for Health Care Facilities*, provides criteria (Sections 4-3.1.2.1 through 4-3.1.2.3 for Type I systems, and Section 4-3.2 for Type II systems).

2. For storage of *gas cylinders* used in health care laboratories, Section 4-3.3.2 of NFPA 99-1987, *Standard for Health Care Facilities*, provides criteria.

3. For storage of *nonflammable gas cylinders* used in nonflammable anesthetizing locations and in administering respiratory therapy in any health care facility, Sections 4-3.1.2.1 through 4-3.1.2.3 of NFPA 99-1987, *Standard for Health Care Facilities*, provides criteria.

4. For storage of *flammable anesthetizing agents* used in flammable anesthetizing locations in hospitals, Section 4-3.1.2.4 of NFPA 99-1987, *Standard for Health Care Facilities*, provides criteria.

5. For storage of *nonflammable gas cylinders* used in nonflammable anesthetizing locations in ambulatory health care facilities, 4-6.2.1.2 of NFPA 99-1987, *Standard of Health Care Facilities*, provides criteria.

Nuclear Material Storage. Many health care facilities utilize radioactive material routinely. Its safe storage is vital since in fires or explosions such material can cause serious side effects for staff, as well as for fire service personnel, in the vicinity. NFPA has developed a document on the subject, NFPA 801-1986, *Rec-

ommended Fire Protection Practice for Facilities Handling Radioactive Materials. Section 4-4 therein contains recommendations with regard to the storage of such material.

Identification of Hazardous Material Being Stored. Knowing the type and level of hazard of the material, liquid, gas, etc., being stored is extremely helpful to fire fighters. To that end, NFPA has developed a sign by which fire service personnel can quickly assess the general hazard level of what is being stored-within. It is the "704" diamond, as outlined in NFPA 704-1985, *Standard System for the Identification of the Fire Hazards of Materials.* The four quarters of the diamond are used to indicate health, flammability, self-reactivity (stability), and special information.

3-6.2. On-Going Activities.

Several locations of on-going activities, including those presenting electric shock hazards, have been identified by NFPA Committees as needing more attention than others. These are:

1. Inhalation anesthetizing locations — hospitals.
2. Patient care areas of hospitals (including anesthetizing locations).
3. Hyperbaric and hypobaric facilities.
4. Laboratories.
5. Non-medical areas.

The fixed localized firesafety systems developed for these areas, and references for them, will be discussed. (These areas, of course, include the building-wide systems discussed previously in Sections 3-4 and 3-5 of this compendium.)

(1) Inhalation Anesthetizing Locations.

Because of the critical nature of activities performed in anesthetizing locations, either localized systems are installed to provide levels of safety above that in other patient care areas, or there are more stringent requirements for any localized systems provided in these areas. These include:

Electric Wiring. Performance criteria are included in 3-4.1.2.1(e) of NFPA 99-1987, *Standard for Health Care Facilities;*

installation requirements are included in Part G of Article 517 of NFPA 70-1987, *National Electrical Code.*

Isolated power systems and line isolation monitors (where installed). Performance criteria are included in 3-4.3 and 12-4.1.3.2 of NFPA 99-1987, *Standard for Health Care Facilities*; installation requirements are included in Part G of Article 517 of NFPA 70-1987, *National Electrical Code.*

Conductive Flooring (where installed). Performance criteria are included in 12-4.1.3.8(b) of NFPA 99-1987, *Standard for Health Care Facilities.*

Piped Gases. (See 3-5.3(1) in this *Compendium.*)

Piped Vacuum. (See 3-5.3(2) in this *Compendium.*)

(2) Patient Care Areas of Hospitals (including anesthetizing locations).

Fire protection for most of the fixed systems in intensive care units, general in-patient care units, and out-patient care areas is included in the building-wide system protection discussed previously in Sections 3-4 and 3-5 of this *Compendium.* Two localized systems that are installed, and for which criteria has been developed, are:

Electric Wiring. Performance criteria are included in 12-3.3.1 of NFPA 99-1987, *Standard for Health Care Facilities*; installation requirements are included in Parts F and G of Article 517 of NFPA 70-1987, *National Electrical Code.* For those areas meeting the definition of *wet location*, paragraph 3-4.1.2.6 in NFPA 99 provides criteria for the type of localized system which has to be installed to provide additional electrical safety.

Isolated power systems and line isolation monitors (where installed). Paragraph 3-4.3 of NFPA 99-1987, *Standard for Health Care Facilities*, includes criteria when such systems are installed; installation requirements for such systems are included in Part G of Article 517 of NFPA 70-1987, *National Electrical Code.*

(3) Hyperbaric and Hypobaric Facilities.

Carrying out procedures under either a compressed atmosphere or non-atmosphere is accomplished in chambers bearing the names hyperbaric and hypobaric, respectively. These facilities present fire hazards because of the increased oxygen content that occurs (sometimes deliberately) within them or within the air being supplied to persons in them.

For hyperbaric facilities, Section 19-2 of NFPA 99-1987, *Standard for Health Care Facilities*, provides criteria on housing and fabrication, ventilation, illumination, fire protection, and electrical systems.

For hypobaric facilities, Chapter 3 of NFPA 99B-1987, *Standard for Hypobaric Facilities*, provides corresponding criteria to those for hyperbaric facilities.

(4) Laboratories.

Guidance on systems in these areas generally can be found in Chapters 5 and 10, of NFPA 99-1987, *Standard for Health Care Facilities*. This includes:

Fire protection in general — 10-5

Electrical outlets — 3-4.1.3

Fume hood protection — 5-4.4 and 5-6.2

Ventilation — 5-4.3

For other laboratories not covered by NFPA 99, NFPA 45-1986, *Standard on Laboratories Using Chemicals* is applicable. Criteria on fire protection systems are contained in Chapter 4, and ventilating systems in Chapter 6 of that document.

(5) Non-Medical Areas.

For non-medical areas, fixed localized firesafety systems, and criteria for them, are the same as can be found in many commercial operations. These include:

(a) Computer Areas: Criteria on facility construction, fire extinguishment, air conditioning, and electrical systems are contained in NFPA 75-1987, *Standard for the Protection of Electronic Computer/Data Processing Equipment.*

(b) Kitchen Areas: These areas present very distinct fire hazards because of the fuels used and the heat generated. Guidance on fixed localized systems include the following:

- For vapor removal (hoods, ducts, grease removal, fire extinguishment, and air movement), NFPA 96-1987, *Standard for the Installation of Equipment for the Re-*

moval of Smoke and Grease-Laden Vapors from Commercial Cooking Equipment, has been developed.

- For gas cooking equipment, Section 6.5 of NFPA 54-1984, *National Fuel Gas Code*, contains criteria.

(c) Waste Disposers: The collection of combustible materials for removal purposes presents a fire hazard because of the unknown condition of the material so collected. There are two methods used to remove waste, and NFPA has developed criteria for each:

- Incineration: Domestic and commercial/industrial incinerators are covered in Chapter 2 of NFPA 82-1983, *Standard on Incinerators, Waste and Linen Handling Systems and Equipment.*

- Compactors: Domestic and commercial/industrial compactors are covered in Chapter 5 of NFPA 82.

3-7. Emergency Communication Systems.

Notifying occupants in a building of an emergency is an obvious necessity. Whatever method is used, if it is to be effective, it must be sufficiently loud or visible to gain the attention of occupants, and it must be almost instinctively associated with an emergency requiring occupants to move or possibly be moved. Whether the medium is a signal or a verbal statement, the conveyance of the emergency must be clear.

An NFPA Committee studied this situation for several years and developed two documents for the two different methods that can be used (a signal or a verbal statement). It was a difficult task because it required consideration of human behavior, language differences, physical limitations, and local traditions. For health care facilities, there was the added dimension of a portion of the occupants in a condition that would preclude any movement in an emergency.

One document is NFPA 72F-1985, *Standard for the Installation, Maintenance, and Use of Emergency Voice/Alarm Communication Systems.* This document contains requirements for speakers used for emergency communications as well as for alarm signals. For voice communication, this could be recorded message and/ or live messages. This type of notification is typically used in high-rise buildings where evacuation of the total building is not feasible or possible or necessary.

The other document developed is NFPA 72G-1985, *Guide for the Installation, Maintenance and Use of Notification Appliances for Protective Signaling Systems*. This document contains recommendations for mounting and locating audible and visual indicating appliances, such as bells, horns, chimes, strobes. Criteria for loudness of these devices is also included. This type of notification is more typically used where evacuation of occupants is anticipated.

NFPA 101-1985, *Life Safety Code*, leaves optional the medium of conveyance of a fire emergency in patient care areas of health care facilities, as long as it is automatic, and does not rely solely on staff. Whatever method is used, however, must be acceptable to the authority having jurisdiction.

Chapter 4   **Operational Fire Protection (Safe Practices)**

In Chapter 3, various types of fire protection that are built into a structure were discussed, with references provided. In this chapter, fire protection necessitating active or continuous involvement by health care personnel in order to be effective will be discussed. For purposes of discussion, this involvement will be termed "operational" fire protection action since it includes safe practices that should be observed at all levels in order to help assure (1) a firesafe working environment for patients and staff; and (2) safe egressing should it be necessary during an emergency.[12] This chapter also includes the maintenance and testing of built-in systems (discussed in Chapter 3) in order to keep such systems functioning properly.

Material in this chapter will be presented in terms of *area*. While this has resulted in some duplication, it was considered the best way to present material. It has been this author's experience that most people trying to find a specific reference are usually aware of the general area in which to look.

The concluding section of this chapter (Section 4-10) will discuss the resources available when a fire situation occurs and some emergency type action is required. However, it should be remembered that response to emergencies will vary for each facility, and that a total emergency plan that takes these variations into consideration needs to be developed.

The *areas* of health care facilities have been categorized for purposes of discussion, as follows:

Section 4-1   Inhalation anesthetizing locations of hospitals

   4-2   Inhalation anesthetizing locations of ambulatory care facilities

   4-3   Patient care areas of hospitals

   4-4   Patient care areas of clinics and ambulatory health care facilities

   4-5   Patient care areas of nursing homes

   4-6   Patient care areas of hyperbaric and hypobaric facilities

   4-7   Laboratories

In addition to the above *areas*, three other categories have been identified:

   4-8   Systems and Their Maintenance

   4-9   Employee Safety—Electrical

   4-10   Emergency Activities (all areas of health care facilities)

4-1. Inhalation Anesthetizing Locations of Hospitals.

Activities in these areas for which safe practices have been developed include the following:

4-1.1. Administration and Maintenance.

(1) All anesthetizing locations: 12-4.1.1.4 and 12-4.1.1.5 of NFPA 99-1987, *Standard for Health Care Facilities.*
(2) Flammable anesthetizing locations: 12-4.1.3.9 of NFPA 99-1987, *Standard for Health Care Facilities.*

4-1.2. Testing of line isolation monitors (Where Installed): 3-5.2.5 of NFPA 99-1987, *Standard for Health Care Facilities.*

4-1.3. Testing of Conductive Floors (Where Installed)

(1) Flammable anesthetizing locations: 12-4.1.3.8(b) of NFPA 99-1987, *Standard for Health Care Facilities.*

4-1.4. Use of Conductive Footwear (Flammable Anesthetizing Locations Only): 12-4.1.3.8(g) of NFPA 99-1987, *Standard for Health Care Facilities.*

4-1.5. Antistatic Testing (Flammable Anesthetizing Locations): 12-4.1.3.8(f) of NFPA 99-1987, *Standard for Health Care Facilities.*

4-1.6. Use of Gas Cylinders, High Pressure:

(1) Safe practices: 4-3.1.1 and 4-6.2.1 of NFPA 99-1987, *Standard for Health Care Facilities*; CGA Pamphlet P-2, *Characteristics and Safe Handling of Medical Gases.*[13]

(2) Color coding: CGA Pamphlet C-9, *Standard Color Marking of Compressed Gas Cylinders Intended for Medical Use in the United States.* Color coding, however, is secondary to labeling of cylinders with the name of the gas contained therein.

(3) Non-interchangeability of fittings for different gases in cylinders: CGA Pamphlet V-5, *Diameter-Index Safety System*, and CGA Pamphlet V-1, *Compressed Gas Cylinder Valve Outlet and Inlet Connections.*

4-1.7. Use of Anesthetic Apparatus:

(1) All anesthetizing locations: 8-5.1.2.1 of NFPA 99-1987, *Standard for Health Care Facilities.*

(2) Flammable anesthetizing locations: 12-4.1.3.8(d) and (e) of NFPA 99-1987, *Standard for Health Care Facilities.*

4-1.8. Use of Electrical Appliances (Line Voltage and Low Voltage):

(1) All anesthetizing locations: 7-5.1.2.2 of NFPA 99-1987, *Standard for Health Care Facilities.*

(2) Flammable anesthetizing locations: 7-5.1.2.4 of NFPA 99-1987, *Standard for Health Care Facilities.*

(3) High-frequency appliances:

Safe use — Annex 2, Safe use of High-Frequency Electricity in Health Care Facilities, of NFPA 99-1987, *Standard for Health Care Facilities.*

Flammable anesthetizing locations — 12-4.1.3.9(j) of NFPA 99-1987, *Standard for Health Care Facilities.*

4-2. Inhalation Anesthetizing Locations of Ambulatory Health Care Facilities.

Activities in these areas for which safe practices have been developed include the following:

4-2.1. Administration and Maintenance: Section 13-4.1.4.3 of NFPA 99-1987, *Standard for Health Care Facilities.*

4-2.2. Use of Anesthetic Apparatus: 13-4.1.2.8 of NFPA 99-1987, *Standard for Health Care Facilities.*

4-3. Patient Care Areas of Hospitals (Including Anesthetizing Locations).[14]

Activities in these areas for which safe practices have been developed include the following. (Note: for non-fixed (portable) devices, testing may actually be performed in non-patient care areas.)

4-3.1. Electrical Safety Program: Section 12-2.5 of NFPA 99-1987, *Standard for Health Care Facilities.* Also, the "Functional Safety and Sanitation Section" of the Joint Commission on Accreditation of Hospitals's *Accreditation Manual for Hospitals* (1984).

4-3.2. Testing of Electrical Grounding System: 3-5.2.1 of NFPA 99-1987, *Standard for Health Care Facilities.*

4-3.3. Testing of Electrical Receptacles: 3-5.2.2 of NFPA 99-1987, *Standard for Health Care Facilities.*

4-3.4. Testing of Ground Fault Circuit Interrupters: 3-5.2.3 of NFPA 99-1084, *Standard for Health Care Facilities.*

4-3.5. Patient Care-Related Electrical Appliances:

(1) Manufacturer requirements: Section 9-2.1 of NFPA 99-1987, *Standard for Health Care Facilities.*

(2) Electrical testing program: Section 7-5.1.3 of NFPA 99-1987, *Standard for Health Care Facilities.*

(3) High-frequency type: Annex 2, Safe Use of High-Frequency Electricity in Health Care Facilities, of NFPA 99-1987, *Standard for Health Care Facilities.*

4-3.6. Use of Oxygen.

Major portions of the material in Chapter 8, Gas Equipment, of NFPA 99-1987, *Standard for Health Care Facilities*, are directed toward safe practices when respiratory therapy is administered (e.g., eliminating sources of ignition, handling cylinders, use of electrical equipment, rules on smoking and sparking toys, etc.). NFPA has also developed a document which describes the problems and hazards created within an oxygen-enriched atmosphere. NFPA 53M-1985, *Manual on Fire Hazards in Oxygen-Enriched Atmospheres*, contains information on the fundamentals of ignition, on materials, on the design of systems, and on the extinguishment of fires in such atmospheres. It also includes a compilation of fires and explosions in which elevated levels of oxygen were present.

4-4. Patient Care Areas of Ambulatory Care Facilities.

Criteria for activities in these areas generally follow those listed in Section 4-3 of this *Compendium*, particularly 4-3.5(b) relative to patient care area appliances.

4-5. Patient Care Areas of Nursing Homes.

Very few national standards have been developed to date for activities in nursing homes. The only specific safe practices are those for respiratory therapy, as provided in Chapter 8, Gas Equipment, of NFPA 99-1987, *Standard for Health Care Facilities*.

4-6. Patient Care Areas of Hyperbaric and Hypobaric Facilities.[15]

4-6.1. Criteria on safe practices in hyperbaric (atmosphere under pressure) facilities are included in Chapter 19, Hyperbaric Facilities, of NFPA 99-1987, *Standard for Health Care Facilities*. Safe practices for equipment handling gases, electrical and electrostatic integrity, and maintenance are discussed in Section 19-3 of that chapter.

4-6.2. Criteria on safe practices in hypobaric facilities (i.e., where the atmosphere has been removed) are listed in NFPA 99B-1987, *Standard for Hypobaric Facilities*. Safe practices for equipment, denitrogenation, handling gases, electrical and electrostatic integrity, and maintenance are discussed in Chapter 5 of that manual.

4-7. Laboratories.

4-7.1. Criteria on safe practices in these areas are contained in Chapters 5 and 10 of NFPA 99-1987, *Standard for Health Care Facilities.* Covered are the following:

1. Maintenance and Inspection: Section 10-8

2. Hazard Assessment: 10-2.2.1

3. Orientation and Training: 10-2.2.1

4. Flammable Liquids (transfer, handling, and disposal): 10-7.4 and 7-7.5

5. Gases: Section 4-3.3.

4-7.2. Guidance on identifying hazardous areas through the posting of a standardized sign is covered in NFPA 704-1985, *Standard System for the Identification of Fire Hazards of Materials.*

4-7.3. Criteria on other activities that can create hazards in laboratories can be found in the following NFPA documents, the titles of which are indicative of the material contained therein.

(1) NFPA 491M-1986, *Manual on Hazardous Chemical Reactions.* This is a listing of approximately 3550 documented chemical reactions.

(2) NFPA 325M-1984, *Fire Hazard Properties of Flammable Liquids, Gases and Volatile Solids.* This is a compilation on the properties of over 1500 flammable liquids, etc.

(3) *Flash Point Index of Trade Name Liquids,* SPP-51 (1978). An alphabetical listing of the flash point of over 8800 products by trade name.

4-7.4. Laboratories not included within the scope of NFPA 99-1987, *Standard for Health Care Facilities,* can find safe practices in NFPA 45-1986, *Laboratories Using Chemicals.* Included in that document are the following:

1. Chemical Storage, Handling, and Waste Disposal: Chapter 7

2. Laboratory Operations: Chapter 9

3. Hazard Identification: Chapter 10.

4-8. Systems and Their Maintenance.

4-8.1. Almost all the systems discussed in Sections 3-4 and 3-5 of this *Compendium* require periodic maintenance and/or testing in order to assure their satisfactory operation, particularly those that operate only in an emergency. To assist readers, a reiteration of systems and where references on maintenance and testing for them can be found is listed below:

(1) Automatic Fire Detectors: Chapter 8 of NFPA 72E-1987, *Standard on Automatic Fire Detectors.*

(2) Smoke Alarms: Chapter 6 of NFPA 74-1984, *Standard for the Installation, Maintenance and Use of Household Fire Warning Equipment.*

(3) Signal Systems for "processing" Signals from Detectors:

Section 1-5 of Chapter 1 in NFPA 72B-1986, *Standard on Auxiliary Protective Signaling Systems.*

Sections 2-3 and 2-4 of Chapter 2 in NFPA 72C-1986, *Standard on Remote Station Protective Signal Systems.*

Section 2-3 and 2-4 of Chapter 2 in NFPA 72D-1986, *Standard on Proprietary Protective Signaling Systems.*

(4) Sprinkler Systems: NFPA 13A-1987, *Recommended Practice for the Care and Maintenance of Sprinkler Systems.*

(5) Fire Hoses: NFPA 1962-1987, *Standard for the Care, Use and Maintenance of Fire Hose*, including connections and nozzles.

(6) Fire Pumps: NFPA 20-1987, *Standard for the Installation of Centrifugal Fire Pumps:*

Turbine type: Sections 4-6 and 4-7 of Chapter 4

High-rise building type: Section 5-6 of Chapter 5

Diesel type: Section 8-6 of Chapter 8

General acceptance, operation, and maintenance: Chapter 11.

(7) Carbon Dioxide Extinguishing Systems: NFPA 12-1985, *Standard on Carbon Dioxide Extinguishing Systems:*

General inspection, maintenance and instruction: Section 1-11 of Chapter 1

Hand hose line systems training: Section 4-6 of Chapter 4

Standpipe system and mobile supply training: Section 5-5 of Chapter 5.

(8) Halon Type Extinguishing System: Section 1-11 of Chapter 1 in NFPA 12A-1985, *Standard on Halon 1301 Fire Extinguishing Systems.*

(9) Dry Chemical Type Extinguishing Systems: NFPA 17-1985, *Standard for Dry Chemical Extinguishing Systems:*

General inspection, maintenance, and instruction: Section 2-10 of Chapter 2

Hand hose line system training: Section 5-6 of Chapter 5.

(10) Piped Gas Systems (Non-Medical Usage): Part 4 (inspection, testing, and purging) of NFPA 54-1984, *National Fuel Gas Code.*

(11) Piped Gas Systems (Medical Usage): Section 4-5 of NFPA 99-1987, *Standard for Health Care Facilities.*

(12) Piped Vacuum Systems (Medical-Surgical Usage): Section 4-9 of NFPA 99-1987, *Standard for Health Care Facilities.*

(13) Normal Electrical System: Section 3-5 of NFPA 99-1987, *Standard for Health Care Facilities:*

Grounding Systems in Patient Care Areas — 3-5.2.1

Receptacles in Patient Care Areas — 3-5.2.2

GFCIs in Patient Care Areas — 3-5.2.3

Isolated Power Systems (where installed) — 3-5.2.5

(14) Essential Electrical System: Section 3-5 of NFPA 99-1987, *Standard for Health Care Facilities.*

Alternate Power Source and Transfer Switches — 3-5.1.2.3

Circuitry — 3-5.1.2.4

Batteries — 3-5.1.2.5

Maintenance Guide — Appendix C-3.2

4-8.2. Some sterilizers use ethylene oxide, a flammable agent, as the sterilizing agent. Guidance on the storage and handling of this product can be found in Section 2-5 of AAMI EO-VRSU, "Good Hospital Practice: Ethylene Oxide Gas — Ventilation Recommendations and Safe Use."[16]

4-9. Employee Safety — Electrical.

Health care facilities have a responsibility for creating and maintaining a reasonably safe environment not only for patients but also for employees. The federal agency established to monitor employees safety is the Occupational Safety and Health Administration (OSHA). Among many areas of concern is that of employee electrical safety; and NFPA has developed a document on the subject, NFPA 70E-1983, *Standard for Electrical Safety Requirements for Employee Workplaces*. NFPA 70E, derived from NFPA 70, *National Electrical Code*, currently provides criteria on both installation safety and work practice safety as they relate to electrical installations in buildings, mobile homes, parking lots, etc.

4-10. Emergency Activities (All Areas of Health Care Facilities).

Health care facilities owners have to be concerned about fire emergencies, just like any other owner of an occupied (or unoccupied) structure. However, because health care facilities are places where people can be brought for treatment, owners have to be concerned not only about emergencies within their facilities, but also with emergencies that might occur near their facilities. Thus, this section is divided into two parts:

4-10.1 Internal emergencies.

4-10.2 External emergencies.

4-10.1. Internal Emergencies.

Each health care facility has to consider its own situation for handling emergencies, be it a small fire in a trash can, a large fire in a storage room, or chemical spill in a laboratory. Factors in preparing and responding to emergencies include the facility's distance from the nearest fire station, the condition of patients, the yearly climatic conditions experienced, the type of training provided to staff, and the construction of the building. All enforcing authorities that this author is aware of, in fact, require facilities to develop a fire response (disaster) plan.

4-10.1.1. Facility-Wide Response.

NFPA has developed criteria for fire situations involving more than one area or a large portion of a facility. Considered internal disasters, such situations would set in motion the facility's internal disaster response plan. In addition to fires, this plan would be activated by such occurrences as bomb threats, the collapse of a building or a portion of one, or the loss of regular and emergency power. Section 1-3 of Annex 1 of NFPA 99-1987, *Standard for Health Care Facilities*, outlines the basic considerations in planning for any type of disaster. Section 1-6 of Annex 1 of NFPA 99 describes a sample plan for internal disaster planning purposes.

For hospitals, the Joint Commission on Accreditation of Hospitals' *Accreditation Manual for Hospitals* (1986) details under Plant, Technology and Safety Management what JCAH expects hospitals, ambulatory health care facilities, long term health care facilities, hospices, and psychiatric, alcoholic, drug-abuse, and mentally retarded/developmentally disabled patient facilities to include in an internal disaster plan.

Larger health care facilities, such as those having multiple buildings or several high-rise buildings, can increase their fire response capability through the creation of staff fire brigades. These are teams of personnel who have been given advanced fire service training in the use of self-contained breathing apparatus, hand lines, etc. NFPA has developed a document, NFPA 600-1986, *Recommendations for Organization, Training and Equipment of Private Fire Brigades*, which provides criteria on training, drills, equipment, and inspection for facilities that create brigades. However, such brigades should not be viewed as substitutes for the regular fire dept.

4-10.1.2. Specific Area Response.

NFPA has developed guidance on internal emergencies for the following areas within a facility:

(1) Anesthetizing locations: Appendix C-12.4 of NFPA 99-1987, *Standard for Health Care Facilities*, contains suggested procedures in the event of a fire or explosion.

(2) Respiratory therapy areas (where oxygen, etc., is being administered for respiratory purposes as opposed to anesthetizing

purposes): Appendix C-8-3 of NFPA 99-1987, *Standard for Health Care Facilities*, contains suggested procedures in the event of a fire associated with respiratory therapy.

(3) Laboratories: (a) general emergency procedures are listed in 10-2.2.3 of NFPA 99-1987, *Standard for Health Care Facilities*; (b) recommendations on body drenching or eye flushing are contained in 10-6 of the same document.

(4) Hyperbaric facilities: (a) Fire involving multiple-occupancy chambers: Appendix C-19.2 of NFPA 99-1987, *Standard for Health Care Facilities*, recommends actions for fires occurring both inside or outside such chambers; (b) Fires involving single-type occupancy chambers: Appendix C-19.3 of NFPA 99-1987, *Standard for Health Care Facilities*, recommends actions for fire occurring both inside or outside such chambers.

(5) Hypobaric facilities: (a) Fire inside a chamber: Appendix C-2.1 of NFPA 99B-1987, *Standard for Hypobaric Facilities*, provides recommendations for this situation; (b) Fire outside a chamber: Appendix C-2.2 of NFPA 99-1987, *Standard for Hypobaric Facilities*, provides recommendations for this situation.

4-10.2. External Emergencies.

Health care facilities also have to be concerned about disasters that occur outside their facilities. These can be natural disasters (e.g., hurricanes, volcanoes, floods, forest fires), as well as human-generated disasters/accidents (e.g., train crashes, release of toxic chemicals in large amounts, civil disturbances, major building fires). All these activities can place a severe strain on health care facility operations; however, if and when they occur, a facility must be prepared for either (1) an influx of large numbers of new patients, (2) an orderly evacuation of current patients as well as health care facility personnel, or (3) a combination of both of these possibilities.

Section 1-3 of Annex 1 of NFPA 99-1987, *Standard for Health Care Facilities*, discusses how a health care facility can prepare for any of these possibilities. As for internal disasters, Section 1-5 of Annex 1 in NFPA 99 provides a sample plan for external disaster planning purposes.

In addition, the Joint Commission of Accreditation of Hospitals' *Accreditation Manual for Hospitals* (1986) details what it expects hospitals to include in an external disaster plan.

For those health care facilities located near airports, inclusion in the airports' emergency plan is very probable. To understand where health care facilities fit into such plans, NFPA 424M-1986, *Manual for Airport/Community Emergency Planning*, may be reviewed. While most of the document is devoted to airport authority activities, knowing such details will help health care facilities understand how they can support airports when an accident or incident involving many victims occurs.

Chapter 5   **Portable Fire Extinguishment Equipment**

A discussion on portable fire extinguishment equipment is included in this *Compendium* because health care facilities require such equipment as part of their fire response capability.[17] Which type is best suited for a particular situation or facility? This should be answered only by a knowledgeable fire protection engineer who can properly analyze a facility's needs, capability, and even location, with regard to the type and extent of deployment of portable fire extinguishment equipment.

5-1. Hand-Held or Wheeled Fire Extinguishers.

There are basically three types of hand-held or wheeled fire extinguishers:

- Liquid (e.g., water, water-based, soda acid, foam)
- Gaseous (e.g., carbon dioxide, Halon)
- Dry chemical.

Each extinguishes a fire using a different principle (e.g., smothering, saturation, oxygen elimination). NFPA has developed a document for such equipment, NFPA 10-1984, *Standard for Portable Fire Extinguishers*. This document provides the following criteria:

1. Categorizes fires into four classes, based on the type of flammable or combustible material involved,

2. Rates fire extinguishers by their ability to extinguish fires according to established test configurations,

3. Classifies fire hazards by the magnitude of fire that can be expected (low, moderate, high),

4. Lists selection criteria,

5. Suggests distribution criteria (how many fire extinguishers should be available based upon area, hazard, and hoses available in a structure),

6. Contains inspection, maintenance, and recharging criteria for extinguishers, and

7. Includes an extensive appendix supplementing the criteria in the text.

In addition to NFPA 10, the 16th edition of the NFPA *Fire Protection Handbook* devotes Section 20 entirely to portable fire extinguishing equipment.

In larger or more remote facilities, large extinguishers, basically the same as described above, are sometimes stationed at strategic points within the facility. Because of their weight, these extinguishers are mounted on wheels in such a way as to make moving them easy while at the same time to make tipping them over extremely difficult.

5-2. Other Portable Extinguishment Equipment.

There are other types of "portable" extinguishment equipment that can be used for extinguishing fires. However, references containing performance features or criteria are much less extensive than for those types just discussed.

5-2.1. Fire Blankets.

Blankets have been used on fires for many decades, but to date no standard has been written on them. Guidance on their use is limited but is included in the following publications:

1. Appendix A-10-2.2.3.3 of NFPA 99-1987, *Standard for Health Care Facilities.*

2. Chapter 4 of Section 20, NFPA *Fire Protection Handbook* (16th Edition).

Reports of a radically different material and procedure for fire blankets have been received at NFPA indicating that technology is being applied to the construction of fire blankets.

5-2.2. Surrounding Material.

A large towel, a regular blanket, a curtain, a scatter rug—fire extinguishers? Yes. There is no standard for their use as fire extinguishers per se, but, with a little training, people can learn how to use them effectively on small fires (such as might occur in a basket or when a person's clothes catch fire) when a regular fire extinguisher is not readily available.

Appendix A   **Agencies or Organizations with an Interest in Health Care Facilities and Firesafety**

As an assistance to readers, the names, addresses, and general activities of a few organizations involved in firesafety and health care facilities are listed below. An extensive listing can be found in the 16th edition of the NFPA *Fire Protection Handbook.*

A-1. Federal Government Agencies.

A-1.1. Center for Fire Research, National Bureau of Standards, Department of Commerce, Washington, DC 20234.

Conducts research in all phases of fire prevention, including studies on human behavior. The Center also developed the Fire Safety Evaluation System (FSES) for health care facilities. It is a method of measuring equivalencies of protection for requirements listed in NFPA 101, *Life Safety Code.*

A-1.2. Federal Emergency Management Agency, 500 C Street SW, Washington, DC 20472.

Responsible for overall coordination of disasters that are considered or designated national in impact. The Agency includes health care facilities in their disaster planning program.

A-1.3. Department of Health and Human Services, Washington, DC 20857.

As the Federal Government third-party payer of hospital and medical charges, the Department utilizes firesafety standards as a means of assurance that the facility it is reimbursing has a particular level of firesafety.

A-2. Non-Government Organizations.

A-2.1. American Health Care Association, 1200 15th Street, NW, Washington, DC 20005.

Has a standing committee on Life Safety which reviews documents on life safety and physical plants. In addition, ACHA has representative on NFPA Technical Committees.

A-2.2. American Hospital Association, 840 N. Lake Shore Drive, Chicago, IL 60611.

Sponsors the American Society for Hospital Engineering which has a committee on codes and standards. This committee reviews codes and standards affecting hospitals, including those covering firesafety documents. In addition, AHA has representatives on many NFPA Technical Committees.

A-2.3. Joint Commission on the Accreditation of Healthcare Organizations, 875 Michigan Avenue, Chicago, IL 60611.

Accredits hospitals, ambulatory health care, and long term care facilities, hospices, and psychiatric, alcoholic, drug abuse and mentally retarded/developmentally disabled patient facilities. Criteria used for accreditation include (1) meeting JCAHO established firesafety criteria, and (2) operating in ways to reduce fire hazards.

A-2.4. National Fire Protection Association, Batterymarch Park, Quincy, MA 02269.

In addition to the development of all types of firesafety documents, including many expressly for health care facilities, NFPA sponsors seminars, develops audio/visual material for use in health care facilities, and has formed a Health Care Section for NFPA members who have an interest in health care firesafety.

A-2.5. National Smoke, Fire and Burn Institute, 90 Sargent Road, Brookline, MA 02146.

Advocate for public firesafety education, including medical staff. Produces films and conducts research.

Appendix B   **Standards Writing Organizations**

Many organizations produce standards that include, either in whole or in part, provisions on firesafety. The methods by which these organizations produce standards vary, so readers should contact each to learn about the procedures used.

The following is a limited list of those organizations whose standards are utilized in whole or in part, either voluntarily or through enforcement, by health care facilities.

B-1. National Fire Protection Association, Batterymarch Park, Quincy, MA 02269.

The NFPA is the oldest and largest developer of voluntary standards on firesafety in the United States. About 60 of the 270 plus documents it develops relate in some way to health care facilities.

B-2. American National Standards Institute, 1430 Broadway, New York, NY 10018.

While the American National Standards Institute (ANSI) does not develop standards itself, it is the national coordinator of voluntary standards development in the United States.

B-3. Occupational Safety and Health Administration, Department of Labor, Washington DC.

This agency produces or adopts standards that are intended to make the workplace a safe environment, including safety from fire.

B-4. Fire Prevention Codes.

Fire prevention codes have been written by many voluntary organizations including the following:

Fire Prevention Code, American Insurance Association, 85 John St., New York, NY 10038.

National Fire Prevention Code, Building Officials and Code Administrators International (BOCA), 4051 West Flossmoor Road, Country Club Hills, IL 60477-5795.

Uniform Fire Code, International Conference of Building Officials (ICBO), 5360 South Workman Mill Road, Whittier, CA 90601.

NFPA 1, Fire Prevention Code, National Fire Protection Association, Batterymarch Park, Quincy, MA 02269.

Standard Fire Prevention Code, Southern Building Code Congress International, Inc., 900 Montclair Road, Birmingham, AL 35213

B-5. Joint Commission on Accreditation of Healthcare Organizations, 875 North Michigan Ave., Chicago, IL 60611.

This non-government accrediting organization has developed an *Accreditation Manual for Healthcare Organizations*, which includes standards on life safety, firesafety, and fire and disaster planning for hospitals, ambulatory health care facilities, long term care facilities, hospices, and psychiatric, alcoholic, drug abuse, and mentally retarded/developmentally disabled patient facilities.

B-6. Compressed Gas Association, 1235 Jefferson Davis Hwy., Arlington, VA 22202.

CGA develops a wide range of standards and recommended practices on the use, markings, etc. for flammable and nonflammable gases.

Appendix C   **Laboratories Testing for Firesafety**

There are many laboratories that can and will evaluate a product or design with respect to firesafety integrity. Many of the tests are applicable to both health care and other types of facilities (e.g., tests for fire doors; tests for insulation for steel beams; tests for electrical receptacles). Other tests, however, would be of interest only to health care facilities (e.g., firesafety tests for X-ray machines). Testing laboratories are operated by the federal government, by universities, and by private owners (either manufacturers or independent operators).

It is the authority having jurisdiction, however, who will advise a facility which testing laboratories' label or listing it will accept on products or materials to be installed in his or her jurisdiction.

Readers should also remember that laboratories test an initial sample and/or a unit from a production run in determining if the product meets a particular standard. This means that a particular unit arriving at a facility has not, in all probability, been subjected to the tests of the standard. However, it does mean that, given good manufacturing practices, the unit is the same as the one tested, and that if the sample passed the test, the unit purchased would also.

Readers can request of testing laboratories the tests to which a product was subjected.

Appendix D   NFPA Documents Cited in This Compendium

NFPA 1, *Fire Prevention Code* (1987)

NFPA 10, *Portable Fire Extinguishers* (1984)

NFPA 12, *Carbon Dioxide Extinguishing Systems* (1985)

NFPA 12A, *Halon 1301 Fire Extinguishing Systems* (1985)

NFPA 13, *Installation of Sprinkler Systems* (1987)

NFPA 13A, *Care and Maintenance of Sprinkler Systems* (1987)

NFPA 14, *Standpipe and Hose Systems* (1986)

NFPA 17, *Dry Chemical Extinguishing Systems* (1985)

NFPA 20, *Centrifugal Fire Pumps* (1987)

NFPA 22, *Water Tanks for Private Fire Protection* (1984)

NFPA 24, *Installation of Private Fire Service Mains and Their Appurtenances* (1984)

NFPA 30, *Flammable and Combustible Liquids Code* (1987)

NFPA 31, *Installation of Oil Burning Equipment* (1987)

NFPA 45, *Fire Protection for Laboratories Using Chemicals* (1986)

NFPA 50, *Bulk Oxygen Systems at Consumer Sites* (1985)

NFPA 53M, *Fire Hazards in Oxygen-Enriched Atmospheres* (1985)

NFPA 54, *National Fuel Gas Code* (1984)

NFPA 58, *Liquefied Petroleum Gases, Storage and Handling* (1986)

NFPA 70, *National Electrical Code* (1987)

NFPA 70E, *Electrical Safety Requirements for Employee Workplaces* (1983)

NFPA 71, *Central Station Signaling Systems* (1987)

NFPA 72A, *Local Protective Signaling Systems* (1987)

NFPA 72B, *Auxiliary Protective Signaling Systems* (1986)

NFPA 72C, *Remote Station Protective Signaling Systems* (1986)

NFPA 72D, *Proprietary Protective Signaling Systems* (1986)

NFPA 72E, *Automatic Fire Detectors* (1987)

NFPA 72F, *Emergency Voice/Alarm Communication Systems* (1985)

NFPA 72G, *Notification Appliances for Protective Signaling Systems* (1985)

NFPA 72H, *Testing Procedures for Protective Signaling Systems* (1985)

NFPA 74, *Household Fire Warning Equipment* (1984)

NFPA 75, *Protection of Electronic Computer/Data Processing Equipment* (1987)

NFPA 78, *Lightning Protection Code* (1986)

NFPA 80, *Fire Doors and Windows* (1986)

NFPA 80A, *Protection from Exposure* (1987)

NFPA 82, *Incinerators, Waste and Linen Handling Systems and Equipment* (1983)

NFPA 85A, *Prevention of Furnace Explosions in Fuel-Oil and Natural Gas-Fired Single Burner Boiler-Furnaces* (1987)

NFPA 88A, *Parking Structures* (1985)

NFPA 90A, *Air Conditioning and Ventilating Systems* (1985)

NFPA 90B, *Warm Air Heating and Air Conditioning Systems* (1984)

NFPA 91, *Blower and Exhaust Systems, Dust, Stock and Vapor Removal or Conveying* (1987)

NFPA 96, *Removal of Smoke and Grease Laden Vapors from Commercial Cooking Equipment* (1987)

NFPA 99, *Health Care Facilities* (1987)[18]

NFPA 99B, *Hypobaric Facilities* (1987)[19]

NFPA *101, Life Safety Code* (1985)

NFPA 211, *Chimneys, Fireplaces, Vents, and Solid Fuel Burning Appliances* (1984)

NFPA 220, *Types of Building Construction* (1985)

NFPA 231, *Indoor General Storage* (1987)

NFPA 231C, *Rack Storage of Materials* (1986)

NFPA 232AM, *Archives and Record Centers* (1986)

NFPA 251, *Standard Methods of Fire Tests of Building Construction and Materials* (1985)

NFPA 255, *Method of Test of Surface Burning Characteristics of Building Materials* (1984)

NFPA 325M, *Fire Hazard Properties of Flammable Liquids, Gases, Volatile Solids* (1984)

NFPA 418, *Rooftop Heliport Construction and Protection* (1979)

NFPA 424M, *Airport/Community Emergency Planning* (1986)

NFPA 491M, *Hazardous Chemical Reactions* (1986)

NFPA 600-1986, *Private Fire Brigades* (1986)

NFPA 704, *Identification of the Fire Hazards of Materials* (1985)

NFPA 801, *Facilities Handling Radioactive Materials* (1986)

NFPA 1961, *Fire Hose* (1987)

NFPA *1962, Care, Maintenance and Use of Fire Hose* (1987)

Flash Point Index of Trade Name Liquids, SPP-51 (1978)

Notes

1. The term "the Association" will mean NFPA throughout the text.

2. Copies available from NFPA.

3. In this section, use of the term "systems" refers to those that utilize stationary components (such as sprinklers, piping, CO_2 tanks, etc.). Portable fire extinguishers will be discussed in Chapter 5.

4. These systems are less extensive than sprinkler or standpipe systems, but can be used in much the same way.

5. Copies of articles can be obtained from the Library of NFPA.

6. Available from either the American Gas Association, 1515 Wilson Blvd., Arlington, VA, 22209, or the American National Standards Institute, 1430 Broadway, New York, New York, 10018.

7. Chapter 4 of this *Compendium* addresses fire and shock hazard from electricity on a different level: operational.

8. There are nine chapters in the 1987 *National Electric Code*. Within each chapter, there are subchapters called articles.

9. Performance, maintenance, and testing criteria for localized electric systems are listed in the next section (Section 3-6) of this *Compendium*.

10. Available from the American Society of Mechanical Engineers, 345 East 47th St., New York, NY 10017.

11. It should be remembered that these systems are in addition to any building-wide fire protection that many be built into the area.

12. The alert reader might ask about the inclusion of "manual" fire extinguishment systems in Chapter 3 (i.e., standpipe systems). Since such systems (even though manual) are building-wide, it was considered more appropriate to include them in Chapter 3 than in Chapter 4.

13. All CGA pamphlets are available from the Compressed Gas Association, 1235 Jefferson Davis Hwy., Arlington, VA 22202.

14. This section (covering all patient scare areas in general) overlaps with Section 4-1; but the requirements of each are not in conflict. A general rule, in applying standards, and applicable in this instance, is that the specific governs over the general. (Conversely, if there is no specific, then the general governs.)

15. Including any anesthetizing locations in the facilities. See Footnote 14.

16. Available from the Association for the Advancement of Medical Instrumentation, 1901 North Fort Myer Drive, Arlington, VA 22209.

17. While this subject is related to the fire extinguishment systems discussed in 3-4.2 of this *Compendium*, it was considered more helpful to discuss portable extinguishers separately since, though mounted on walls or in cabinets, they are used only when removed from their fixed locations.

18. NFPA 99 incorporated (and thus replaced) the following documents: NFPA 3M *Health Care Emergency Preparedness* (1980); 56A *Use*

of Inhalation Anesthetics (1978); 56B *Respiratory Therapy* (1980); 56C *Laboratories in Health-Related Institutions* (1980); 56D *Hyperbaric Facilities* (1982); NFPA 56F, *Nonflammable Medical Gas Systems* (1983); 56G *Use of Inhalation Anesthetics in Ambulatory Care Facilities* (1980); 56HM *Home Use of Respiratory Therapy* (1982); 56K *Medical-Surgical Vacuum Systems in Hospitals* (1980); 76A *Esssential Electrical Systems for Health Care Facilities* (1977); 76B *Safe Use of Electricity in Patient-Care Areas of Hospitals* (1980); 76C *Safe Use of High-Frequency Electricity in Health Care Facilities* (1980).

19. NFPA 99B was formerly part of NFPA 99 for 1984 edition. Prior to that it was a separate document, designated NFPA 56E. It was made a separate document again for 1987 because such facilities are no longer utililzed for medical purposes.

Appendix E
Health Care Fire Safety Checklist
Burton R. Klein, MSE

[The following checklist will be useful to readers. It provides a broad overview of the fire protection systems that have to be considered when building a health care facility.]

During the design and construction of a health care facility, an architect or builder will periodically stop for a moment to see if the design will meet the code or the work is going according to plan. Usually, this means checking over a list of items to make sure that nothing has been forgotten.

Several types of lists may be used for this purpose, including an exterior facility design checklist, an interior design checklist, and the traditional "punch list" used during a final inspection. However, none of these has a separate heading specifically for fire protection features.

To fill this gap, the following Fire Protection Checklist for Health Care Facilities has been drawn up. It is based on the NFPA's *Health Care Facilities Compendium — 1984*, which deals with both facility and operational fire protection requirements. Starting with the location of the building and the area around it, the compendium covers both general and specific facility fire protection requirements for a health care institution. For operational fire protection requirements, the compendium is organized by systems and location.

The Fire Protection Checklist for Health Care Facilities should be used during the planning stages of a project to help the architect make sure that the necessary fire protection features have been incorporated into the building design. The builder should also use it during construction to make sure that none of the fire protection requirements has been neglected. As construction draws to a close, the builder or even the owner may want to consult the list again, just to make certain that nothing has been overlooked.

Reprinted with permission from NFPA, *Fire Journal*, Vol. 79, No. 4, Copyright © 1985, National Fire Protection Association, Quincy, Mass. 02269.

Readers are warned that no one checklist can be all-encompassing. Health departments in each state have their own firesafety requirements, as do state building codes. In addition, some localities have adopted the firesafety recommendations contained in the U.S. Department of Health and Human Services' *Guidelines for Construction and Equipment of Hospital and Medical Facilities*. And finally, the requirements for alterations to an existing facility will differ significantly from those for a new high-rise, in-patient, multi-purpose medical center. Thus the specific firesafety requirements of all agencies or organizations having authority over a health care facility should be determined before the design is finalized. If they are not included in this checklist, they should be added to it.

Health Care Facility Fire Protection Checklist

When using the checklist, examine each entry to see whether it is applicable to the project at hand. When the checklist is completed, every entry should have a check mark next to it.

To use the checklist, obtain copies of the documents shown in parentheses after each applicable entry. Given the number of NFPA documents that may pertain, it might be economical to have on hand a set of the NFPA's *National Fire Codes*, which contains a copy of all NFPA documents.

When all the documents needed for a particular project have been collected, review the document that appears in parentheses after each applicable entry. In some instances, an entire document will have to be examined. In others, however, only portions of the document will apply. To help locate relevant portions more quickly, the *Health Care Facilities Compendium* can be used.

When the checklist has been completed, any entries marked "No" will have to be addressed, either directly or through equivalencies acceptable to the authorities having jurisdiction.

Since the NFPA is unaware of any similar checklist, readers are invited to comment on the list to help us improve it and make it as useful as possible. Please direct any comments to Burton R. Klein, Health Care Firesafety Specialist, NFPA, Batterymarch Park, Quincy, MA 02269.

Fire Protection Checklist for Health Care Facilities

	Meets the Requirements		Not Applicable
	Yes	No	

I. Facility Fire Protection

A. Location of Building

1. Adjacent buildings' hazard levels (state building codes) | | | |
2. Fire exposure (NFPA 80A) | | | |

B. Area Around Building

1. Bulk storage of flammable gases (NFPA 30, 50, 58)
2. Bulk storage of flammable liquids (NFPA 30, 50, 58)
3. Bulk storage of non-flammable (oxidizing) gases (NFPA 30, 50, 58)
4. Bulk storage of non-flammable (oxidizing) liquids (NFPA 30, 50, 58)
5. External water supplies (tanks) for fire protection (NFPA 22)
6. Hydrants (NFPA 24)
7. Incinerators/compactors (NFPA 82)
8. Fire lanes (NFPA 1)
9. Parking garages (NFPA 80)

C. Structural Protection

1. Chimneys, fireplaces, etc. (NFPA 211)
2. Flame spread of finish materials (NFPA 101, 251, 255)
3. Floor-ceiling assemblies (NFPA 101)
4. General construction protection (NFPA 101; building codes)
5. Laboratories in health care facilities (HFC) (NFPA 99, Chapter 7)
6. Lightning protection (NFPA 78)
7. Rooftop heliport (NFPA 418)
8. Separation of mixed occupancies (NFPA 101)

233

Fire Protection Checklist (*continued*)

	Meets the Requirements		Not Applicable
	Yes	No	
I. Facility Fire Protection			
9. Solid-fuel-burning appliances (NFPA 211)	||	||	||
10. Walls (NFPA 101)	||	||	||
11. Windows and doors (NFPA 101, 80)	||	||	||
D. Life Safety Considerations			
1. Building services (NFPA 101, Chapter 7)	||	||	||
2. Construction features (NFPA 101, Chapters 5 & 6, NFPA 220)	||	||	||
3. Exit access/exits/exits discharge (NFPA 101, Chapter 5)	||	||	||
4. Fire protection (NFPA 101, Chapter 7)	||	||	||
5. General health care requirements (NFPA 101, Chapters 12/13)	||	||	||
6. Handicapped provisions (each state, either in the building code or separate legislation)	||	||	||
7. High-rise consideration (NFPA 101)	||	||	||
8. Laboratories in HCF (NFPA 99, Chapter 7)	||	||	||
9. Operating features (NFPA 101, Chapter 31)	||	||	||
E. Detection/Extinguishment Systems			
1. Detection systems (NFPA 101, 72 series, 74)	||	||	||
2. Extinguishment systems (NFPA 101, 12, 12A, 13, 13A, 14, 17)	||	||	||
F. Other Fire Protection Equipment			
1. Fire pumps (NFPA 20)	||	||	||
2. Hoses (NFPA 1961, 1962)	||	||	||
G. Fixed Building-Wide Service Systems			
1. Fuels for heating systems			
Bases (NFPA 54)	||	||	||
Liquids (NFPA 30)	||	||	||

2. Heaters
   Gas (NFPA 54, ANSI Z83.3, NFPA 85A)
   Oil (NFPA 31, 85A)
3. Air movement/restrictions (fire and smoke dampers) (NFPA 90A, 90B)
4. Electrical service
   Normal (NFPA 70, 99, Chapter 9)
   Emergency (NFPA 70, 99, Chapter 8)
5. Specific Building Services
   Chutes (waste, linen, etc.) (NFPA 82, 101)
   Elevators/escalators (ANSI/ASME A17.1, NFPA 101)
   Fans (NFPA 91)
   Piped gas systems (flammable) (NFPA 54)
   Piped gas systems (nonflammable) (NFPA 56F)
   Piped gas systems (labs, HCF) (NFPA 99, Chapter 7)
   Piped gas systems (non-HCF labs) (NFPA 45)
   Piped vacuum systems (med-surg) (NFPA 99, Chapter 6)

H. Fixed, Localized Systems
1. Storage areas
   Flammable liquids (NFPA 30, 99)
   Gases (NFPA 56F, 99)
   General (NFPA 231)
   Historical data (NFPA 232C)
   Identifying hazard level (NFPA 704)
   Nuclear material (NFPA 801)
   Rack (NFPA 231C)
2. For anesthetizing locations (NFPA 99, Chapter 3, 4)
3. For other patient care areas (NFPA 99, Chapter 9)
4. For laboratories in HCF (NFPA 99, Chapter 7)
5. For compactors (NFPA 82)
6. For computer areas (NFPA 75)

Fire Protection Checklist *(continued)*

| | Meets the Requirements | | Not Applicable |
| | Yes | No | |

7. For kitchens (NFPA 96, 54) | __ | __ | __ |
8. For hyperbaric facilities (NFPA 99, Chapter 10) | | | |

II. Operational Fire Protection
A. Systems and Their Maintenance
1. Automatic fire detectors (NFPA 72E) | __ | __ | __ |
2. Emergency electric power systems (NFPA 99, Chapter 8) | __ | __ | __ |
3. Normal electric power systems (patient care areas) (NFPA 99, Chapter 9) | __ | __ | __ |
4. Other extinguishing systems (NFPA 12, 12A, 17) | __ | __ | __ |
5. Piped gas systems (NFPA 56F, 54) | __ | __ | __ |
6. Piped vacuum systems (med-surg) (NFPA 99, Chapter 6) | __ | __ | __ |
7. Signal systems (for detectors) (NFPA 72 series) | __ | __ | __ |
8. Smoke alarms (NFPA 74) | __ | __ | __ |
9. Sprinkler systems (NFPA 13A) | __ | __ | __ |
B. Other Fire Protection Equipment
1. Fire hoses (NFPA 1962) | __ | __ | __ |
2. Fire pumps (NFPA 20) | __ | __ | __ |
3. Portable fire extinguishers (NFPA 10) | __ | __ | __ |
C. Employee Safety-Electrical (NFPA 70E) | __ | __ | __ |
D. Response to Disasters (internal and external) (NFPA 99, Appendices C & D) | __ | __ | __ |

E. By Location
   1. Anesthetizing location, hospitals (NFPA 99, Chapter 3) |||||||
   2. Anesthetizing location, ambulatory care facilities (NFPA 99, Chapter 4) |||||||
   3. General patient care areas, hospitals (NFPA 99, Chapter 5, Chapter 9)
   4. General patient care areas, nursing homes (NFPA 99, Chapter 5)
   5. Laboratories in health care facilities (NFPA 99, Chapter 7)
   6. Hyperbaric facilities (NFPA 99, Chapter 10)

Note: For corresponding section in 1987 edition of NFPA 99, see cross-reference table in 1987 edition.

Appendix F
Health Care Construction Safety Checklist

The following is a list of guidelines to consider in order to provide a safe work environment on the construction site. It is not intended to replace any mandatory requirements of local, state, or federal agencies. Since each project has its own set of hazards, a reliable and qualified safety consultant should be contacted.

NOTE: This list should not be considered all-inclusive.

1. Is adequate medical attention available, and have instructions been given to employees as to where and how it can be obtained?

2. Are first-aid kits provided and readily available? Is it posted who is available to do various emergency treatments that might be needed?

3. Are emergency phone numbers posted? Is a phone provided from which emergencies can be reported (with no money required)?

4. Are hard hats provided (for both employees and visitors)?

5. Is adequate hearing protection provided that conforms to federal standards?

6. Is eye and face protection provided as needed?

7. Are safety belts provided and in good repair?

8. Is an adequate number of portable fire extinguishers provided with appropriate capacity?
   A. Is a 2A-rated extinguisher provided per 3,000 square feet?
   B. Is a 2A-rated extinguisher within 100 feet of any point on building site?

Based on "Construction Safety Checklist," by Camplin, Bartel & Associates, Inc., Chicago, IL; copyright © 1986.

C. Is a 10B-rated extinguisher within 50 feet of any location having more than 75 gallons of flammable liquid?

D. Are portable extinguishers given a monthly visual inspection, an annual testing, and an adequate hydrostatic test?

E. Do all trucks and mobile equipment have at least one portable extinguisher?

F. Are fire alarm instructions posted near exits and telephones?

G. Are all employees instructed in the use of all types of extinguishers?

9. Have instructions been given in the use of power and hand tools?

A. Are guards provided?

B. Are all power tools grounded or double insulated?

C. Are all power tools in good operating condition?

10. Have adequate instructions been given in the use of welding and cutting tools?

A. Are all valve caps in place when equipment is not in use?

B. Are all cylinders secured?

C. Are all gas hoses in good condition?

D. Are face guards and hand protection provided?

11. Are all scaffolds in good condition?

12. Are all floor and wall openings protected?

A. Are top rails 42 inches high?

13. Are all electrical supply lines in good condition?

A. Are all cords the three-wire grounded type?

B. Are extension cords of adequate rating?

14. Is proper lighting provided throughout work area?

15. Are all pertinent Occupational Safety and Health Administration (OSHA) regulations being used?

16. Has a qualified safety consultant been retained?

Appendix G
Providing Those Other Essential Services
(A Checklist)

This appendix is included to show when the services that are built into a facility need to be considered. Three phases are identified: the design stage, the construction stage, and the post-construction stage. Use of this checklist will vary with the extent of construction and with whether a project is creating a new facility or adding to an existing one.

A. GROUND COVER

A-1. Design Stage. (A follow-up at each level of design and planning must be done.)

a. A complete survey of the property, aimed at indicating all possible problems: topographical, grading, drainage, perimeter land use, roads, ledge, trees, ponds, utility lines (both above and below the ground), walls, walks.

b. A survey of all existing buildings to indicate floor levels, entrances, exits, steps, ramps, equipment floor use (by floor), utility entrances and exits, building materials, window types, and so on.

c. Zoning requirements, easements, right of ways, fire department access.

d. Boring (subsurface) data: test pits should be obtained.

e. Parking probability studies. Roadway access, roadway exit. Public, emergency, outpatient, service and delivery study.

NOTE: All ground cover work has to be done at the design stage.

240

B. ELECTRICITY (NORMAL)

B-1. Design Stage. (Includes all phases of design from initial study to final working drawings.)

a. All electric power information should be verified, for example, location of power sources, those from which power may be obtained, extent of power, need for extra transformers, distance onto public property power lines will need to go, overhead or underground power requirements, responsibility for paying for the line of supply (some or all).

b. Determination early on where entry into building will take place. Allow adequate space for this area.

c. Location and size of fuel storage if electricity is to be generated on site.

B-2. Construction Stage.

a. Caution! Underground lines are not always where they are shown on surveys. Many fatal accidents have occurred because of bulldozers hitting unknown lines. A constant check for this problem must be done.

b. Temporary power and who pays for it (owner, contractor, or both) must be considered.

c. A check of *all* permits is necessary.

d. Ascertain that designed power has ample safety factors as well as capability for future expansion.

e. Inspection of *all* work must be done.

B-3. Postconstruction Stage

a. A final inspection and testing by proper authorities *before* acceptance.

b. An instructional session with contractor and equipment supplier.

c. All records, plans, and instructional data submitted and properly filed.

    d. A competent engineer hired by facility to operate the system.

    e. An approved preventive maintenance check system.

    f. A complete record of daily use initiated for review by inspection authorities, including certificate of approval agency and insurance carrier.

C. ELECTRICAL (EMERGENCY)

C-1. Design Stage. (Includes all phases of planning and drawing.)

    a. Determination of capacity (load). (See Chapter 3 of NFPA 99–1987, *Standard for Health Care Facilities.*)

    b. Determination of equipment needed (consider future needs and activities).

    c. For generator sets, allowance for adequate air supply and exhaust.

    d. If possible, mounting of equipment above flood or any water source.

    e. A check of all local codes for required coverage.

C-2. Construction Stage. Same as for normal power; see B-2.

C-3. Postconstruction Stage. Same as for normal power; see B-3.

D. WATER (DOMESTIC AND FIRE)

D-1. Design Stage.

    a. A check of water sources. At least two separate supplies should be available.

    b. A check of all pressures. For example, at what level above ground can pressure be maintained? What pressure is required?

    c. A check of source pipe size and of needed pipe to size to meet any added requirements. (Many cities and towns have begun to require two separate water lines to a source: one for domestic use and one for fire use. This can be a cost item.)

d. Determination of source of *hot* water for general use, kitchen use, dish washer use, surgical use, and laboratory use.

e. Determination if sprinklers are required.

f. Determination if piped chilled water is required.

g. Determination if water treatment for hard water is required.

h. Check of codes on the use of PVC (polyvinyl chloride) piping.

i. Desirability and possibility of a passive hot water system (i.e., a solar system).

D-2 Construction Stage.

a. The use of temporary water and fire lines must be considered. It must be agreed as to who pays for this service.

b. All underground lines must be tested, inspected, and approved before trenches are filled. All underground lines must be accurately shown on drawings for future use.

c. All systems must be tested and checked for use of silver solder. (Lead solder is not permitted anywhere anymore.)

NOTE: The plumbing contractor, responsible for water, is often also responsible for the sewer and gas systems. See sections E and G, respectively.

D-3. Postconstruction Stage.

a. A complete set of as-built drawings should be produced that indicate all pertinent valves, shut-offs, clean-outs, and so on.

b. A competent engineer should be retained on site to maintain system.

c. A complete set of data (manuals) on all equipment should be obtained.

d. A preventive maintenance program for the system should be provided.

e. A stock of spare parts should be purchased.

f. Approval of system by building and fire departments should be obtained.

g. Approval by the local department of public works should be obtained.

E. SEWAGE (SANITARY AND STORM)

E-1. Design Stage. (Includes *all* design phases.)

a. Determination if system is public or private.

b. Extent of system needed and capacity required to carry drainage (including consideration for overload).

c. Determination of who pays for connection at street.

d. Determination if street lines need added capacity and who will pay for it.

e. Check if separate lines are required for sanitary and storm water. (Many cities and towns have begun to require this separation. Even if they do not have a completed separate system, they may require owners to install a pipe out cap if ["stub out"] to proposed connection.)

f. Determination if a holding pond or roof-holding system for storm water is required (some cities and towns require this). For a roof system, a check of structural requirements will be necessary.

E-2. Construction Stage.

a. Temporary lines must be considered.

b. No trenches are to be filled until systems are tested and approved.

c. All pumps are to be tested.

d. All systems are to be tested and approved by proper authorities.

E-3. Postconstruction Stage.

    a. A complete set of as-built drawing should be produced that indicate exact location of all lines, shut-offs, and so on.

    b. A complete set of files on systems should be established.

    c. A stock of spare parts should be purchased.

    d. A competent engineer should be retained on site to maintain these systems.

F. HEATING, VENTILATING, AIR CONDITIONING (HVAC) AND OTHER ENVIRONMENTAL CONTROLS

NOTE: This is the most complicated of systems from a design standpoint because many factors are involved in maintaining a controlled environment. It is further complicated if it involves tying into an existing system. Further, none of these environmental systems can work independently; each must work to complement the other.

F-1. Design Stage.

    a. Determination of the best systems for use in the particular facility.

NOTE: There are many combinations of methods of obtaining the best end results, such as cold and hot water, cool and hot air, electrical heating, heat pumps, and air exchange systems. The very building itself can affect the requirements, through its wall construction, insulation, window type (number), location of glass), and so on. A complete study by a specialist of *several* systems must be done. Recall that a health care facility is *not* an office building; each space has unique requirements: from exact temperature control to humidity control.

    b. Determination of which fuels are best for the systems selected.

    c. Check of all pertinent codes.

d. Check of fuel storage locations and their capacities.

F-2. Construction Phase.

a. Constant check and test of each system throughout construction phase.

b. Check of all fire dampers and control dampers *before* they are difficult to access. Each needs to be identified for location for future inspection.

c. Check of all fire walls for proper penetration and sealing.

d. Complete inspections by the proper authorities.

F-3. Postconstruction Stage.

a. A complete set of as-built drawings is to be produced for each system.

b. A complete set of data files on equipment is to be provided.

c. A competent engineer should be retained on site to operate and maintain these systems.

d. A preventive maintenance program for each system is to be provided. Tests for each system are to be conducted on a regular basis (depending on manufacturer information and actual use).

e. A daily record of activities and actions is to be kept.

G. GAS AND VACUUM SYSTEMS (MEDICAL)

G-1. Design Stage (All Phases).

NOTE: 1. Gas and vacuum systems are, in most cases, designed by the plumbing and sanitary engineer. 2. Medical gas is a very important design item; accidents have occurred by interconnecting pipes carrying different gases. 3. Medical compressed air is considered a gas like oxygen and nitrous oxide, etc. 4. Piped vacuum systems look like piped gas systems and are installed similarly and simultaneously in many instances; they are different technologies, however, and should be treated accordingly. 5. See Chapter 4 in NFPA 99— 1987, *Standard for Health Care Facilities*, which covers installation and performance criteria for both piped gas and piped vacuum systems.

a. All gas station outlets must be keyed to the different gases they will be carrying. This applies to vaccum station inlets as well.

b. All drawings must be approved by the proper authorities.

c. *Propane gas* for laboratory use must be clearly identified.

d. Location of exterior gas supplies is to be identified early on in site plan studies.

G-2. Construction Stage.

a. Testing of all lines should be done periodically, and not at the end of construction.

b. All pipelines (gas and vacuum) are to be clearly labeled with the gas they will be carrying. Arrows showing direction of flow are to be added at regular intervals. Labeling is to be done as work progresses, not at the end of construction. (Color coding is not the prime method of identification; it can lead to serious errors.)

c. All underground lines are to be tested prior and immediately after trench fill.

d. All lines are to be blown out, cleaned, and tested.

e. All pumps are to be checked. (A standby pump should be considered.)

G-3. Postconstruction Stage.

a. A complete set of as-built drawings is to be provided.

b. A preventive maintenance program for each system is to be provided.

c. A stock of spare parts should be purchased.

H. COMMUNICATION

H-1. Design Stage. (All phases.)

a. Determination early on as to what types of systems are desired and which are possible (e.g., a 12-volt system can include many items besides a telephone, such as intercom, music, doctors' and nurses' call systems, patient call and answer, emergency announcements, data control).

b. Consideration for video (television) should be made since it is a form of communication.

c. Extensive use of computers for patient management, pharmacy control, billing, and environmental control should be planned for. A complete room by room or space by space study of present and future needs should be made.

d. Fire alarms and smoke detection systems are a vital communications link, and their compatibility with decor needs to be considered, too (e.g., proper arrangement on ceilings and walls in conjunction with HVAC outlets and with lighting).

e. In some large facilities, a fire control space is required to coordinate alarms and systems.

f. A check of all codes must be done as required.

g. The devices used for security control are now very diverse and require consideration: television monitors, door alarms, pharmacy alarms, electric eyes, floodlights (e.g., for parking areas, entrances). Some systems will require a space for a person to monitor them.

H-2. Construction Stage.

a. Constant testing and checking during installation.

b. Inspection by proper authorities.

H-3. Postconstruction Stage.

a. A complete set of as-built drawings is to be provided.

b. All panels are to properly and legibly identified and adequately lighted. All circuits are to be labeled. Data are to be filed.

c. A competent engineer is to be retained on site to operate and maintain the systems.

d. A stock of spare parts (e.g., circuit boards) should be purchased.

e. A preventive maintenance program for each system is to be provided by manufacturer or supplier.

f. All items requiring fire department response are to be inspected by the local fire department (a regular inspection schedule should be developed at the first inspection).

A note regarding agencies involved in the preceding stages: Consultation with the proper authorities and knowledge of the codes they use are of primary importance. The following agencies, which are noted elsewhere in this book but are repeated here for emphasis, are some of the more common ones that are encountered during the construction process:

1. Department of Public Health (local, state) — interested in all aspects of the patient and the health of employees in general. Enforces codes and issues certificates to operate a facility.

2. Department of Public Safety (local, state) — interested in the safety of all, with special attention to the handicapped. Enforces codes.

3. Department of Public Utilities (local, state) — interested in the use of all utilities.

4. Department of Health and Human Services (federal, state) — interested in general safety of patients; reimburses facilities for treating Medicare or Medicaid patients; funds research; enforces codes.

5. Fire Department (local, state) — interested in all aspects of fire and/or disasters, including the emergency medical technicians and ambulance use. Enforces codes.

6. Police Department (local, state) — interested in traffic control, access road ingress and egress.

7. Occupational Safety and Health Administration (federal) —interested in all aspects of safety. Very active during construction stage. Uses and enforces standards. Can impose fines for deficiencies and other acts of noncompliance.

8. Certificate of Approval — independent agency interested in review of facility for compliance with health codes and regulations. The facility pays for this service.

9. Environmental Board (local, state, federal) — interested in the control of the environment from problems stemming from water, air, gas, land, swamps, waterways, and pollution of any kind.

10. Planning Department (local) — interested in the control of community density, type of construction, land use. In most cases, it has regulations for the community served.

11. Certificate of Need or Certificate of Determination (local, state, federal). Determines if proposed project can be carried out based on the need for the service(s) to be provided. Associated with federal reimbursement for Medicare and Medicaid patients.

12. Air Traffic Control — interested in air space control (e.g., height of buildings, lights) near airports.

NOTE: Compliance with these agencies is necessary. It should be remembered, though, that many of these agencies have departments under them that may have their own set of approval procedures. Some of these subdepartments include radiology, newborn, laboratory, toxicology, pathology, nursing homes, long-term care, and use of public land.

Glossary

As with any field, there are words of the trade; terms or acronyms that have meaning peculiar to the subject at hand. The following are definitions of the more common terms used throughout this text.

NOTE: These definitions are those of the authors.

Accreditation   A level of operation of a facility deemed acceptable to the organization that inspected the facility.

Approved drawings   Drawings approved by a *specific authority*.

Authority having jurisdiction (AHJ)   Any group, agency, institute, or other organization that enforces codes and standards.

Capital improvements   Improvements of a financial scale and/or physical magnitude as to require various approvals, both within and without the institution.

Certificate of Need (CON)   An authorization to build or renovate a structure within specified bounds and cost. (See Chapter 2.)

Clerk of the works   A person with appropriate training who is hired by the owner as a "watchdog" over the construction of a facility. (See Chapter 14.)

Construction management   A method of construction whereby a contractor (builder) is engaged by the owner early in the design stage to provide hands-on cost analysis from actual experience. The contractor, in most cases, is also the actual builder and may give a guaranteed price prior to completion of the drawings. (See Chapter 14.)

Decking   Flooring or roof structure.

Determination of need (DON)   A method of assessing the actual need to purchase an item or construct anything concerning a health care facility within certain levels. The CON committee that makes the DON will issue a CON after approving the project.

Fast Track   A method of construction that starts construction *prior* to completed drawings. This method is used most often during inflation in order to preorder items and attempt to beat the market.

Licensure   A state health agency's authorization to open a facility and treat patients. Limitations of treatment are always specified.

Prefabricated   A manufactured item that is preassembled before shipment.

Prestressed   A structural item of reinforced concrete that is *manufactured* with stressed reinforcing.

Punch list   A final review list of all items to be completed by the contractor.

Smoke zone   An area within a structure, vertical or horizontal, so separated from other areas as to restrict the passage of smoke.

Turnkey operation   A construction method whereby one firm performs all of the tasks from design to final occupancy, in most cases for a set cost that is included in the entire package.

Bibliography

The following publications are presented as possible sources of additional information. It is not an exhaustive listing and should not be considered as an endorsement by either the authors or the publisher.

ADMINISTRATION

Building a Hospital: A Primer for Administrators, by J. Rea, J. Fromelt, M. MacCoun. Chicago, American Hospital Association, 1978.

Certificate of Need Programs: A Review, Analysis and Annotated Bibliography of the Research Literature. Washington, D.C., U.S. Department of Health, Education, and Welfare, Superintendent of Documents, November 1978, Publication No. (HRA) 79-14006.

Hospital Architecture: Guidelines for Design and Renovation, by D.R. Porter. Melrose Park, Ill., Health Administration Press, 1982.

Hospital-Based Medical Office Buildings, by D. Toland and S. Strong. Chicago, American Hospital Association, 1986.

Hospital Project Financing and Refinancing Under Prospective Payment, by J.L. Elrod, Jr, and J.A. Wilkenson. Chicago, American Hospital Association, 1985.

Hospitals and the News Media: A Guide to Good Media Relations, by M.L. Babich. Chicago, American Hospital Association, 1985.

Planning and Managing Major Construction Projects: A Guide for Hospitals, by D.J. Rohde et al. Melrose Park, Ill., Health Administration Press, 1985.

Status Report on State Certificate of Need Programs. Washington, D.C., U.S. Department of Health and Human Services, Superintendent of Documents, Publication No. (HRP) 0906296.

Suggested Planning Guidelines for SNF/ICF Long Term Care Facilities. Washington, D.C., American Health Care Association, 1974.

Working with Health Care Consultants, by J.G. Nackel et al. Chicago, American Hospital Association, 1986.

ARCHITECTURE

Design Planning for Freestanding Ambulatory Care Facilities, by B. Rostenberg. Chicago, American Hospital Association, 1987.

Designs That Care: Planning Health Facilities for Patients and Visitors, by J.R. Carpman et al. Chicago, American Hospital Association, 1986.

Handbook of Architectural Design Competition. Cat. No. 4J500. Washington, D.C., American Institute of Architects, 1987.

Selection of Architects for Health Facility Projects. Chicago, American Hospital Association, 1975.

Signs and Graphics for Health Care Facilities (An AHA Handbook) Chicago, American Hospital Association, 1978.

Site Selection for Health Care Facilities, by J.G. Lifton and O.B. Hardy. Chicago, American Hospital Association, 1982.

CODES AND STANDARDS

Code Manual for Health Care Facilities, by A.J. Platt. Chestnut Hill, Mass. The Ritchie Organization,

Guide to NFPA National Building Firesafety Standards. Quincy, Mass., National Fire Protection Association, 1983.

Health Care Firesafety Compendium, by B.R. Klein. Quincy, Mass., National Fire Protection Association, 1987. (Reprinted in Appendix D of this book.)

Standards Development in the Private Sector: Thoughts on Interest Representation and Procedural Fairness, by R.G. Dixon, Jr. Quincy, Mass., National Fire Protection Association, 1978.

Model Building Codes

NOTE: Model building codes are updated almost yearly; use depends on which year is adopted in each locale.

National Building Code. Country Club Hills, Ill., Building Officials and Code Administrators International.

Standard Building Code. Birmingham, Ala., Southern Building Officials Congress International.

Uniform Building Code. Whittier, Calif., International Conference of Building Officials Congress International.

CONSTRUCTION

Guidelines for Construction and Equipment of Hospitals and Medical Facilities, 1983/1984 edition. Rockville, Md., U.S. Department of Health and Human Services (PHS, HRSA, Bureau of HMO and Resources Development, Division of Facilities Conversion and Utilization), 1984.

Hospital Based Medical Office Buildings, by D. Toland with S. Strong. Chicago, American Hospital Association, 1981.

Site Selection for Health Care Facilities, by J. Lifton and O. Hardy, Chicago, American Hospital Association, 1982.

Index

skeleton and, 38
utility hookup and, 126

Data storage, 136
Dedication ceremony, 131–33
Defend in place concept of fire
   management, 63, 83
Demolition plans, 100
Department of Defense, 81
Department of Health, Education
   and Welfare, 10
Department of Health and
   Human Services, 222
accreditation and, 126
Certificate of Need and, 10, 13
codes and, 80, 140
*Guidelines for Construction and
   Equipment of Hospitals and
   Medical Facilities,* 68, 84, 232
internal operational
   requirements and, 67
loans from, 16
Department of housing and
   Urban Development, 16
Department of Public Safety, 122
Departments of public health, 125
Design
-build method of construction,
   51–52, 117, 136
codes and, 87–88
development drawings, 94–95
essential services checklist and,
   240, 241, 242–43, 244, 245–48
firesafety checklist and, 231–37
Detection and extinguishing
   systems, 215–16, 234, 236.
   See also Fire; Sprinkler
   systems
Determination of Need (DON), 58
Dietary department, 149, 207–8,
   236
Documentation, 136–38
Drafters, 95–96
Drainage, renovation and, 75
Drawings, 93–105
computer-generated, 95–96
design development, 94–95

fees for, 134
fire inspections and, 122
Mylar overlay, 95–96
review of, 114
scale, 94
storage of, 137
working, 97–104

Electricity, 63–64, 241–42
drawings and, 103
engineers' knowledge of, 46
existing building evaluation
   and, 145
final connections of, 127
firesafety checklist and, 235, 236
laboratories and, 207
NFPA documents concerning,
   198–200, 211, 212, 216–17
patient care areas, 206
sub bids and, 115
wiring installation permit, 113
Elevations, 100–101
Elevators, 63, 69–70
codes and, 86
dedicated, 70
demolition plans and, 100
firesafety checklist and, 235
foundation and, 31
inspections of during
   construction, 120, 122
NFPA documents concerning,
   202
permits for, 113
Emergency
communication systems, 208–9
department, 65–66, 69, 149–50
power, 63–64, 87, 127, 145,
   199–200, 216, 235, 236
Energy conservation, exterior
   renovation and, 75
Engineer, 45–50
changes and, 104, 117
civil, site plan and, 99
drawings and, 94–95, 103–4
evaluation of existing facilities
   and, 59
fees, 134–35

safety during construction and,
123
salvage and, 100
selection of contractor and, 51
signing of approvals by, 126
straight bid construction and,
115–16
utility hookup and, 126
zoning boards and, 24

Parking, 68
essential services checklist and,
240
existing building evaluation, 144
garages, 184, 233
handicapped, 23, 68, 144
location of facility and, 7
renovation and, 76
zoning and, 23
Patient care areas, 71, 212–13,
235, 236
Patients, potential, 29
Payments, 134–36, 137
Percentage fee, 52
Permits, 112–15
Plumbing
drawings and, 95, 102–3
engineers' knowledge of, 46
existing building evaluation, 145
installation permit, 113
sub bids and, 115
Project coordinator, 96
Project manager, 121
Public relations consultant, 107
Public transportation, 7
Punch list, 129

Radio frequency (rf) interference
drawings, 103
Radiology areas, 69, 161
Registered landscape architect, 99
Renovation
architect/engineer fees for, 50
architecture of, 74–77
evaluation of existing facilities
and, 56

inspections and, 122
Mylar overlay drawings and, 97
safety during construction and,
123–24
Research, fund raising and, 17, 18
Revenue, generating, 17–19. See
also Fund raising
Ritchie Organization, The, 67
Roadways, 68
Room finish schedule, 101

Safety during construction,
123–24
Safety inspections, 120–21. See
also Inspections
Scientific Apparatus Makers
Association, 80
Sewage, 128, 244–45
Site plan, 99
Site survey, 99
Size of facility, 4, 5, 37
Size restrictions, 22, 31
Skeleton of building, 37–38
Sketches, 93
Skin of building, 39
Special details drawings, 101
Specification book, 95, 99, 121, 134
Spending money, plan for, 19–21
Sprinkler system, 25, 83, 87–88,
102. See also Fire
Standards, 177, 223–25
Start-up, 125–30
State law
Certificate of Need and, 10
codes and, 84
elevator size, 70
financing and, 15, 16
inheritance, 18
lottery regulations, 18
permits and, 115
safety during construction and,
123
scale drawing requirements
and, 94
taxes and, 15
water conditions, 27